Nuclear Medicine and
Molecular Imaging
Case Review Series

Series Editor

David M. Yousem, MD, MBA
Vice-Chairman Radiology, Program Development
Associate Dean, Professional Development
Department of Radiology
Johns Hopkins School of Medicine
Baltimore, Maryland

Volumes in the CASE REVIEW Series

Nuclear Medicine and Molecular Imaging
Case Review Series

THIRD EDITION

LILJA BJÖRK SÓLNES, MD, MBA
Assistant Professor of Radiology and Radiological Science
Johns Hopkins Medicine
Baltimore, MD

HARVEY ZIESSMAN, MD
Professor of Radiology and Radiological Science
Johns Hopkins Medicine
Baltimore, MD

CONTRIBUTING AUTHOR
SOPHIA T. KUNG, MD
Medical Director
Valley Radiology Imaging
Samaritan Site
San Jose, CA

ELSEVIER

Library of Congress Control Number: 2019935765

Content Strategist: Kayla Wolfe
Content Development Manager: Kathryn DeFrancesco
Content Development Specialist: Caroline Dorey-Stein
Publishing Services Manager: Shereen Jameel
Project Manager: Aparna Venkatachalam
Designer: Amy Buxton

Printed in China

Last digit is the print number: 9   8   7   6   5   4   3   2   1

ELSEVIER

3251 Riverport Lane
St. Louis, Missouri 63043

Working together
to grow libraries in
developing countries

www.elsevier.com • www.bookaid.org

To Rawn, my constant source of strength.
And to Jón, Vivi, and Ari, who make it all worth it.
L.B.S.

Series Foreword

I am so excited about the launch of the third edition of *Nuclear Medicine and Molecular Imaging: Case Review Series*. This topic has been one of the most cherished in the *Case Review Series* and I am gratified to have two renowned physicians (and personal friends here at Hopkins), Lilja B. Solnes MD, MBA and Harvey A. Ziessman, MD, MBA, along with Sophia T. Kung, M.D. as its authors. These are knowledgeable physicians at the forefront of nuclear medicine and molecular imaging who have provided cases that illustrate pathology that one needs to know.

In the nuclear medicine edition there also must be allowance for a large dollop of physics and safety information, part and parcel of handling the radioactive agents. The authors have addressed pathology in all organs of the body and have emphasized techniques, diagnoses, and treatments.

The approach here is unique in that it is case-based and relies on imaging studies to make the teaching points with board review questions and answers for each case, as is the model for the CRS. Congratulations to the authors—and to the readers who will benefit from their wisdom.

David M. Yousem, MD, MBA
Vice-Chairman Radiology, Program Development
Associate Dean, Professional Development
Department of Radiology
Johns Hopkins School of Medicine
Baltimore, Maryland

Contents

Case 1

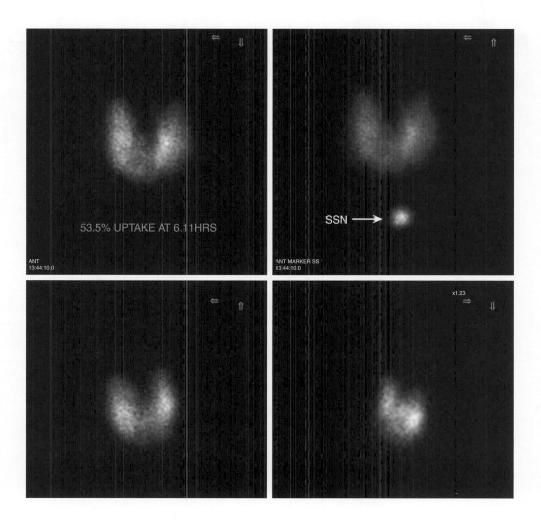

1. What is the most likely diagnosis in this thyrotoxic patient?
   a. Graves' disease
   b. Subacute thyroiditis
   c. Multinodular toxic goiter
   d. Toxic adenoma
2. What is the normal radioiodine uptake range for thyroid scan at 24 hours?
   a. Less than 10%
   b. 15–30%
   c. 30–50%
   d. Greater than 50%

3. What is an appropriate definitive therapy for Graves' disease?
   a. Surgery
   b. Cytomel
   c. Synthroid
   d. I-131 therapy
4. All of the following clinical symptoms are typical for Graves' disease EXCEPT:
   a. Anxiety
   b. Perspiration
   c. Weight loss
   d. Ptosis

Case 2

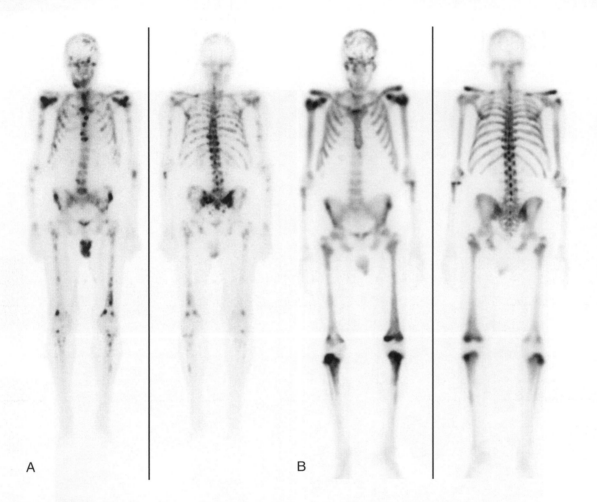

A   B

1. What is your interpretation of the bone scan in this patient with prostate cancer (Image A)?
   a. Disseminated infection
   b. Multiple fractures
   c. Multiple hereditary exostoses
   d. Osseous metastases
2. These lesions are most likely to have what appearance on a concurrent computed tomography (CT) scan?
   a. Blastic lesions
   b. Lytic lesions
   c. Mixed lytic and sclerotic lesions
   d. No CT correlation

3. What other scintigraphic diagnosis can be made on the follow-up bone scan (Image B)?
   a. Degenerative joint disease
   b. Superscan
   c. Penile cancer
   d. Sacral insufficiency fracture
4. What other U.S. Food and Drug Administration (FDA)–approved positron emission tomography (PET) radiopharmaceutical has been approved for evaluation for prostatic metastases?
   a. Indium-111 (In-111)–capromab pendetide
   b. Gallium-68 (Ga-68) DOTA-TATE
   c. Fluorine-18 (F-18) fluciclovine
   d. Ga-67 citrate

Case 3

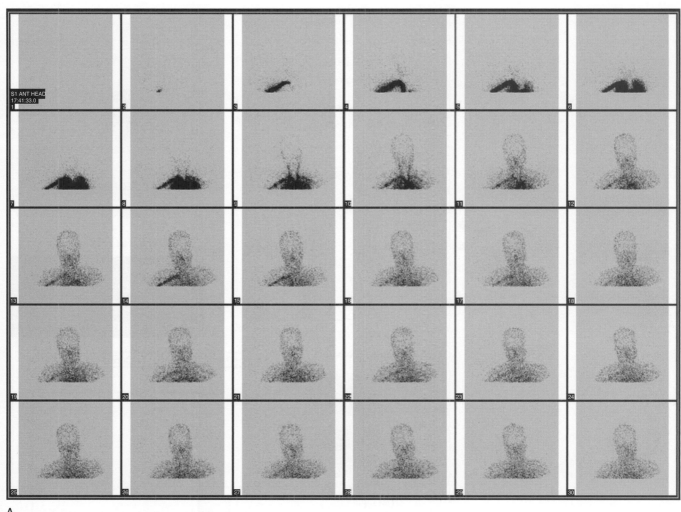

A

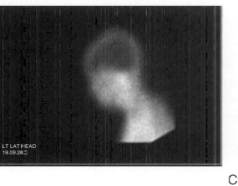

B

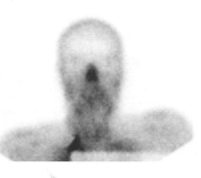

C

1. What is the radiopharmaceutical?
   a. Technetium-99 (Tc-99) dimercaptosuccinic acid (DSMA)
   b. Tc-99 hexamethylpropyleneamine oxime (HMPAO)
   c. Tc-99 red blood cell (RBC)
   d. Tc-99 macroaggregated albumin (MAA)
2. What is your interpretation of this study?
   a. Negative for intracerebral tumor
   b. Negative for osteomyelitis
   c. Brain death
   d. Cerebrovascular territorial infarct
3. The mechanism of this radiopharmaceutical's localization is:
   a. Receptor binding
   b. Polar hydrophilic molecule trapped within neurons
   c. Rapid phosphorylation
   d. Binding to the presynaptic transporter
4. Why do we see increased blood flow to the nose (Figure 3C)?
   a. Upper respiratory infection
   b. Diversion of blood flow from internal to external carotid system
   c. Normal increased vascularity
   d. Increased flow to the nose not seen

Case 4

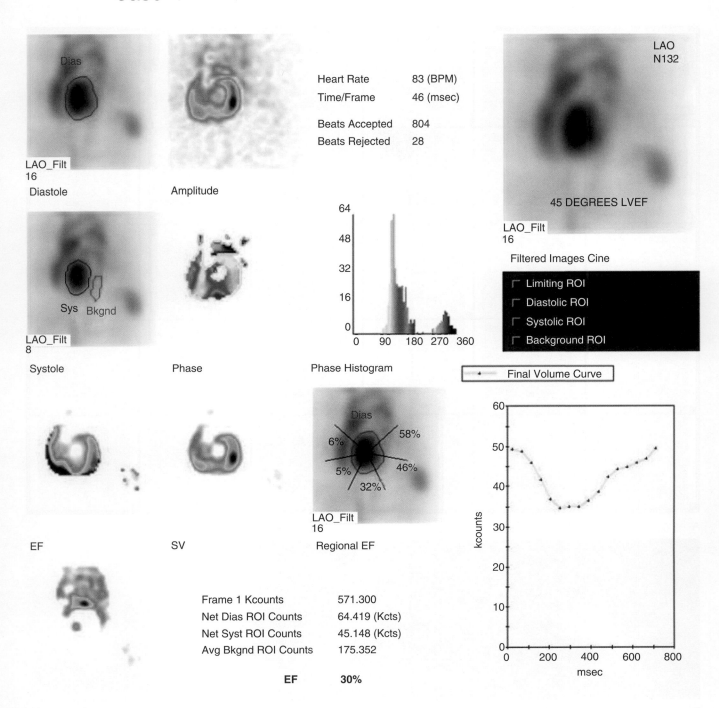

Heart Rate   83 (BPM)

Time/Frame   46 (msec)

Beats Accepted   804

Beats Rejected   28

Diastole

Amplitude

Systole

Phase

Phase Histogram

EF

SV

Regional EF

Filtered Images Cine

- Limiting ROI
- Diastolic ROI
- Systolic ROI
- Background ROI

Final Volume Curve

45 DEGREES LVEF

Frame 1 Kcounts   571.300

Net Dias ROI Counts   64.419 (Kcts)

Net Syst ROI Counts   45.148 (Kcts)

Avg Bkgnd ROI Counts   175.352

EF   30%

1. What is the most common indication for performing a multi-gated acquisition (MUGA) study?
   a. Evaluation for cardiac ischemia
   b. Evaluation for hibernating myocardium
   c. Evaluation of ventricular function
   d. Evaluation for myocardial infarction
2. What view is used to calculate a left ventricular ejection fraction (LVEF)?
   a. Right anterior oblique
   b. Left anterior oblique
   c. Left lateral
   d. Anterior

3. Which radiopharmaceutical is used for the MUGA study?
   a. Tc-99m sestamibi
   b. Tc-99m RBC
   c. Tc-99m human serum albumen
   d. Thallium-201
4. What drug is commonly associated with cardiac toxicity and reduced cardiac function?
   a. Doxorubicin
   b. Zolpidem
   c. Metoprolol
   d. Atorvastatin

Case 5

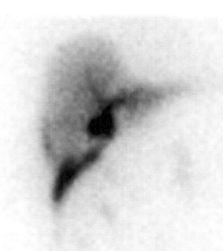

1. What is your interpretation of this Tc-99m hepatobiliary iminodiacetic acid (HIDA) study?
   a. Acute cholecystitis
   b. Hepatitis
   c. Chronic cholecystitis
   d. Biliary leak
2. What is the most likely cause for this problem?
   a. Recent laparoscopic cholecystectomy
   b. Spontaneous gallbladder perforation
   c. Gastric reflux
   d. Biliary fistula

3. What is the incidence of bile leak after cholecystectomy?
   a. Less than 15%
   b. 15–25%
   c. 25–50%
   d. Greater than 50%
4. What is the most common clinical symptom associated with a
   bile leak?
   a. Nausea
   b. Vomiting
   c. Abdominal pain
   d. Palpable mass

Case 6

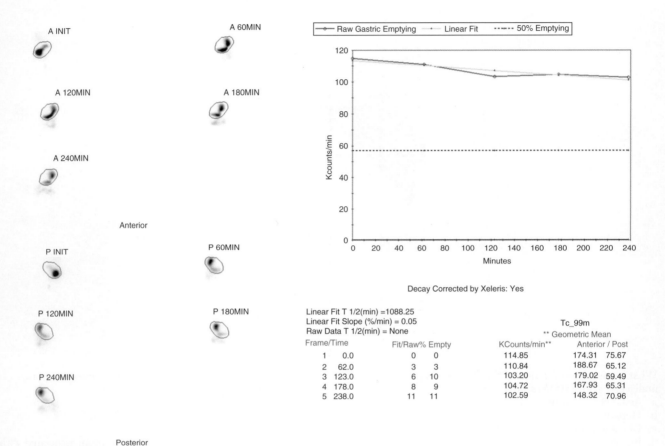

A INIT

A 60MIN

A 120MIN

A 180MIN

A 240MIN

Anterior

P INIT

P 60MIN

P 120MIN

P 180MIN

P 240MIN

Posterior

Legend: Raw Gastric Emptying — Linear Fit ----- 50% Emptying

Decay Corrected by Xeleris: Yes

Linear Fit T 1/2(min) =1088.25
Linear Fit Slope (%/min) = 0.05
Raw Data T 1/2(min) = None

Tc_99m
** Geometric Mean

Frame/Time		Fit/Raw% Empty		KCounts/min**	Anterior / Post	
1	0.0	0	0	114.85	174.31	75.67
2	62.0	3	3	110.84	188.67	65.12
3	123.0	6	10	103.20	179.02	59.49
4	178.0	8	9	104.72	167.93	65.31
5	238.0	11	11	102.59	148.32	70.96

1. This is an example of a very delayed solid gastric emptying study. According to the 2008 Consensus Recommendations for Radionuclide Gastric Emptying Scintigraphy, the standard recommended meal includes:
   a. 4 oz whole egg, 2 slices of toast, strawberry jam (30 g), water (120 mL)
   b. 4 oz egg white, 2 slices of toast, strawberry jam (30 g), water (120 mL)
   c. 4 oz whole egg, 1 slice of toast, Ensure (8 oz mL)
   d. 4 oz egg white, 1 slice of toast, Ensure (8 oz mL)
2. The most sensitive time point for detection of delayed gastric emptying is:
   a. 1 hour
   b. 2 hours
   c. 3 hours
   d. 4 hours
3. The most common cause for chronic functional delayed gastric emptying is:
   a. Diabetes mellitus
   b. Cushing's syndrome
   c. Hyperthyroidism
   d. Zollinger-Ellison syndrome
4. The pattern of solid emptying is:
   a. Exponential
   b. Exponential after a lag phase
   c. Linear
   d. Linear after a lag phase

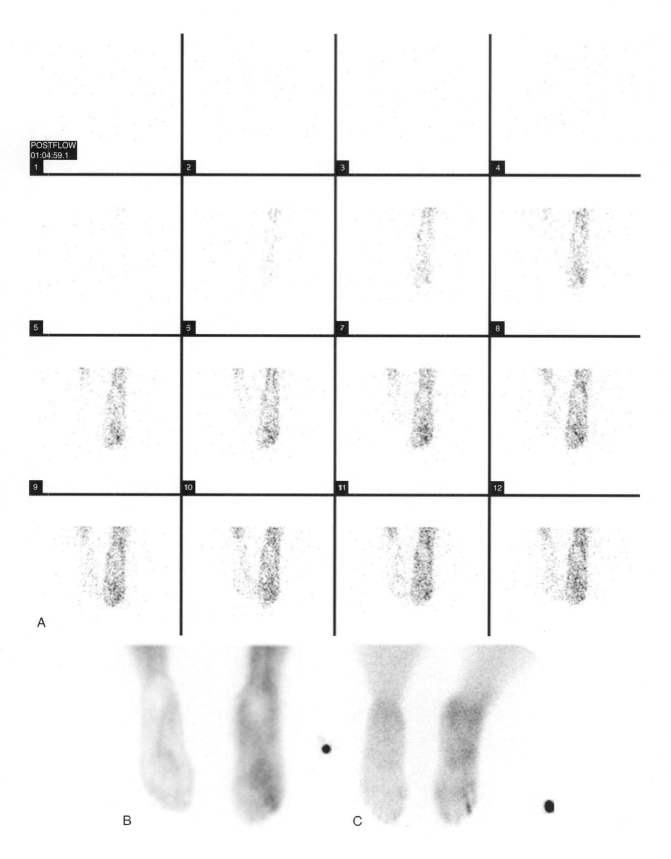

POSTFLOW
01:04:59.1

A

B

C

1. This is a three-phase bone scan consistent with osteomyelitis of the fourth digit of the right foot. In addition to osteomyelitis, what is another common cause for a positive three-phase bone scan?
   a. Cellulitis
   b. Fracture
   c. Edema
   d. Hematoma
2. In the setting of a positive three-phase scan for osteomyelitis, what additional radionuclide test can be ordered to increase specificity?
   a. Tc-99 RBC
   b. Tc-99 pertechnetate
   c. In-111 leukocyte scan
   d. Tc-99 sulfur colloid
3. False-negative studies are uncommon, but may be seen in what age group of patients?
   a. Infants
   b. 2–12 years of age
   c. 20–50 years of age
   d. Greater than 60 year of age
4. What is the most common organism that may cause osteomyelitis?
   a. *Staphylococcus aureus*
   b. *Enterobacter*
   c. *Streptococcus*
   d. *Staphylococcus epidermidis*

Case 8

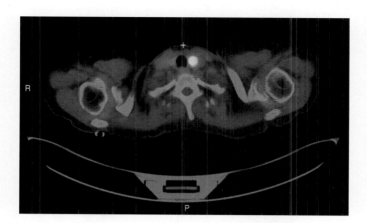

1. What is the pertinent finding?
   a. Focal fludeoxyglucose (FDG) avid lesion in the thyroid gland
   b. FDG avid level 4 adenopathy
   c. Diffuse uptake in the thyroid gland
   d. Vascular inflammation
2. What is the probability of malignancy?
   a. <1%
   b. 5%
   c. 20%
   d. 30%

3. What is the next step?
   a. Ultrasonography (US) and possible tissue sampling
   b. Surgical resection
   c. Ablation
   d. No follow-up needed
4. Which malignancies in the thyroid gland may be FDG avid?
   a. Papillary thyroid cancer
   b. Anaplastic thyroid cancer
   c. Lymphoma of the thyroid gland
   d. All of the above

Case 9

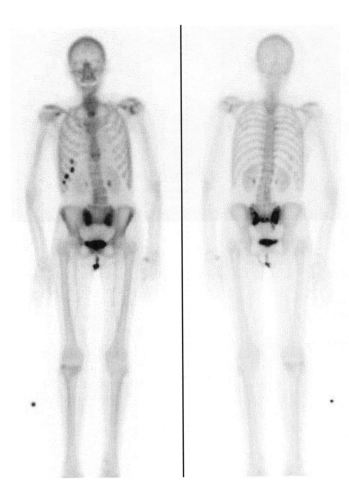

1. What is the best overall interpretation of this bone scan?
   a. Malignant tumor
   b. Normal sacroiliac joint asymmetry
   c. Sacral insufficiency fractures
   d. Degenerative joint disease
2. What was the likely initiating event of the pelvic abnormalities?
   a. Severe trauma
   b. Mild trauma
   c. Infection
   d. Degenerative joint disease

3. The most likely underlying disease process is:
   a. Prostate cancer
   b. Diabetes mellitus
   c. Osteoporosis
   d. Hypertension
4. The most likely treatment plan includes:
   a. Conservative therapy
   b. Open surgery
   c. Chemotherapy
   d. Radiation therapy

Case 10

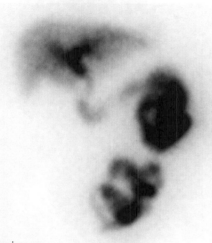

A 1-hour image

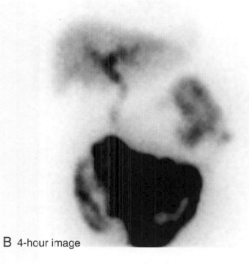

B 4-hour image

1. The mechanism of uptake and excretion of the radiopharmaceutical used to diagnose acute cholecystitis is similar to:
   a. Bilirubin
   b. Albumin
   c. Renin
   d. Cholecystokinin
2. If the gallbladder is not visualized after 60 minutes of imaging, administration of what drug should be considered?
   a. Propranolol
   b. Cholecystokinin
   c. Morphine
   d. Valium
3. What is the above drug's mechanism of action?
   a. Gallbladder contraction
   b. Gallbladder relaxation
   c. Relaxation of the sphincter of Oddi
   d. Constriction of the sphincter of Oddi
4. What is the most frequent cause for cystic duct obstruction?
   a. Stone
   b. Stricture
   c. Bile
   d. Extrinsic compression

Case 11

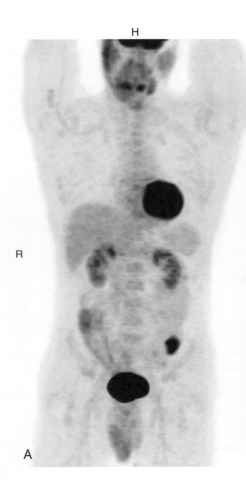

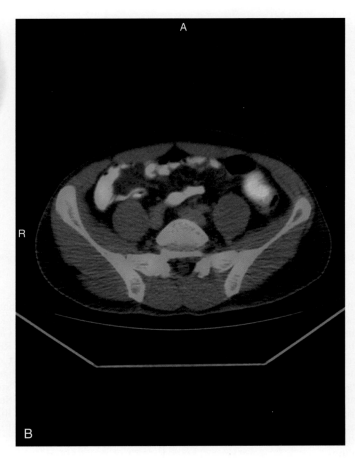

1. What is the likely diagnosis?
   a. Fat necrosis
   b. Colon cancer
   c. Focal diverticulitis
   d. Metastases
2. Focal uptake in what region of the large bowel is thought to be physiologic in the absence of abnormal CT findings?
   a. Ileocecal valve
   b. Hepatic flexure
   c. Splenic flexure
   d. Rectosigmoid
3. What should the serum blood sugar measure before injection of F-18 FDG?
   a. Less than 140 mg/dL
   b. Less than 200 mg/dL
   c. Less than 300 mg/dL
   d. Less than 350 mg/dL
4. How often is incidental focal activity seen in the large bowel on a F-18 FDG PET scan a result of a progressive abnormality?
   a. 90%
   b. 50%
   c. 20%
   d. 10%

Case 12

ANTERIOR   POSTERIOR

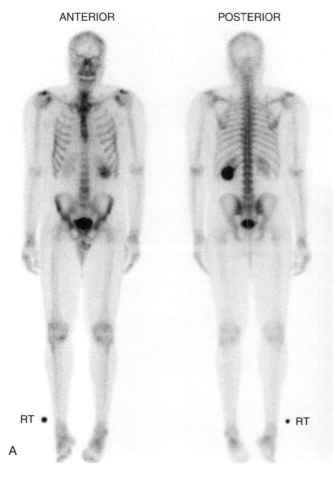

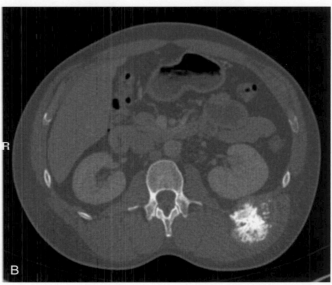

1. The most common primary malignant osseous tumor in children and adolescents is:
   a. Osteosarcoma
   b. Chondrosarcoma
   c. Metastases
   d. Ewing's sarcoma
2. What is the indication for bone scintigraphy with osteosarcoma?
   a. Evaluate for pulmonary metastases
   b. Evaluate for concurrent osteomyelitis
   c. Evaluate extent of primary lesion
   d. Evaluate for skip lesions

3. The most common site for this abnormality in children and adolescents is:
   a. Skull
   b. End of long bones
   c. Pelvis
   d. Ribs
4. The best modality to evaluate the extent of the primary lesion is:
   a. CT
   b. PET/CT
   c. US
   d. Magnetic resonance imaging (MRI)

Case 13

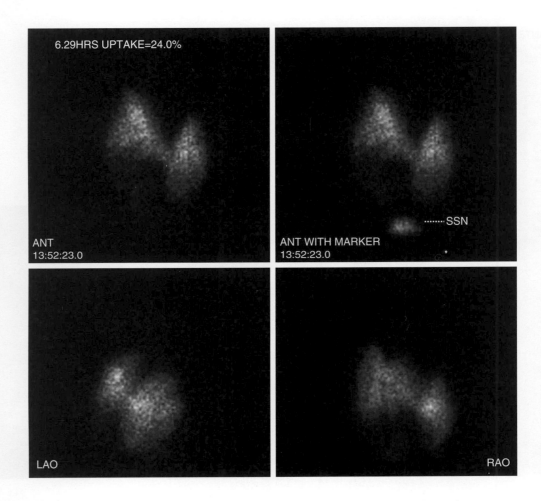

1. Which radiotracer is organified by the thyroid gland?
   a. Tc-99m pertechnetate
   b. I-123
   c. Tc-99m sestamibi
   d. Tc-99m diethylene-triamine-pentaacetate (DTPA)
2. What type of collimator is used for imaging of the thyroid gland?
   a. Pinhole
   b. Parallel hole
   c. Divergent
   d. Convergent
3. What is the next step in management of this patient?
   a. CT scan
   b. Thyroid US
   c. MRI
   d. I-123 whole body (WB) scan
4. What is the likelihood of malignancy?
   a. 1%
   b. 5%
   c. 15%
   d. 30%

Case 14

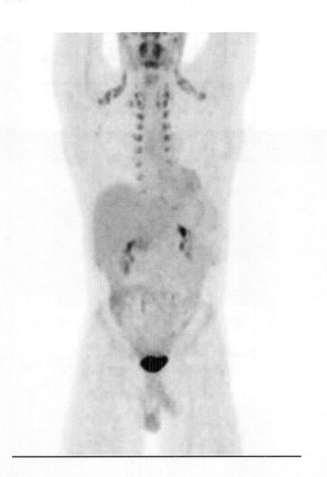

1. What is the most likely cause for F-18 FDG uptake in this patient?
   a. Malignant lymphoma
   b. Brown adipose tissue
   c. Muscle tension
   d. Lymphadenopathy
2. Could any specific patient preparation have been used to minimize this finding?
   a. No
   b. Corticosteroids
   c. Beta blockers
   d. Benadryl

3. In which patients is this finding most likely to be seen?
   a. Children
   b. Men
   c. Women
   d. Elderly
4. What best describes the physiologic function of brown fat activation?
   a. Receptor binding
   b. Parasympathetic autoregulation
   c. Thermoregulation
   d. Fasting

Case 15

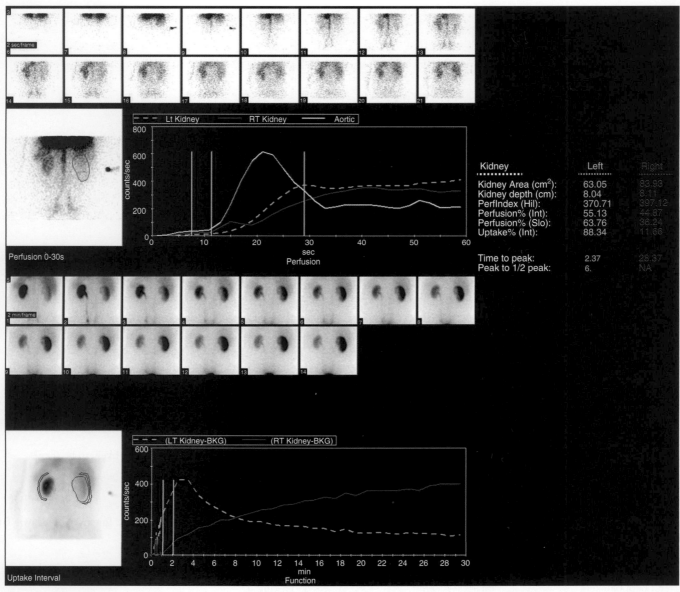

Perfusion 0-30s

Kidney	Left	Right
Kidney Area (cm²):	63.05	83.93
Kidney depth (cm):	8.04	8.11
PerfIndex (Hil):	370.71	397.12
Perfusion% (Int):	55.13	44.87
Perfusion% (Slo):	63.76	36.24
Uptake% (Int):	88.34	11.66
Time to peak:	2.37	28.37
Peak to 1/2 peak:	6.	NA

Uptake Interval

A

1. What is a standard preparation for this study?
   a. Hydration
   b. Beta blocker
   c. Angiotensin-converting enzyme (ACE) inhibitor
   d. Lasix

2. Which radiotracer should be administered when performing a renal function scan in a patient with renal dysfunction?
   a. Tc-99m DTPA
   b. Tc-99m mercaptoacetyltriglycine (MAG3)
   c. Tc-99m DMSA
   d. Tc-99m sulfur colloid

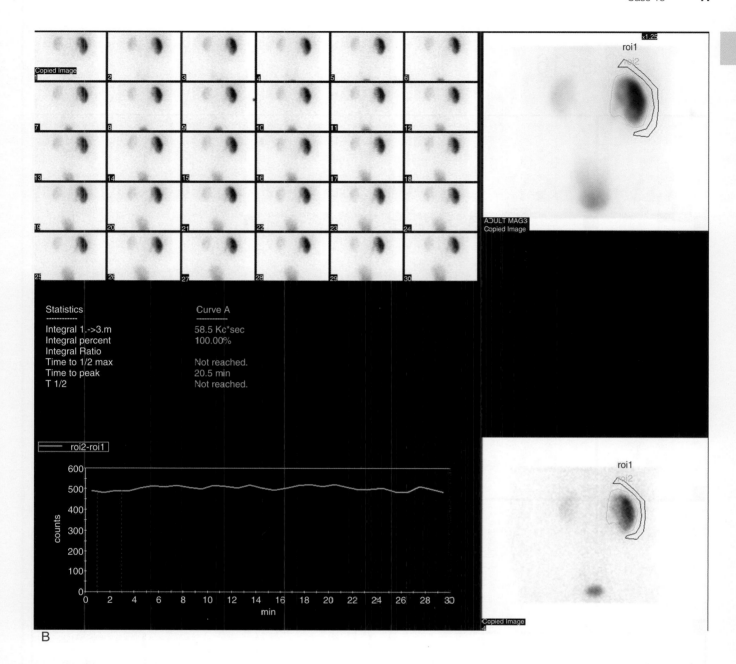

B

3. What is the mechanism of action of Lasix?
   a. Blocking the absorption of sodium, chloride, and water, resulting in increased diuresis
   b. Increasing the absorption of sodium, chloride, and water to increase diuresis
   c. Blocking the absorption of sodium, chloride, and water resulting in decreased diuresis
   d. Increasing the absorption of sodium, chloride, and water to decrease diuresis

4. What half-time (t½) is considered highly suspicious for obstruction (choose the best answer)?
   a. Less than 5 minutes
   b. Less than 10 minutes
   c. Greater than 10 minutes but less than 15 minutes
   d. Greater than 20 minutes

Case 16

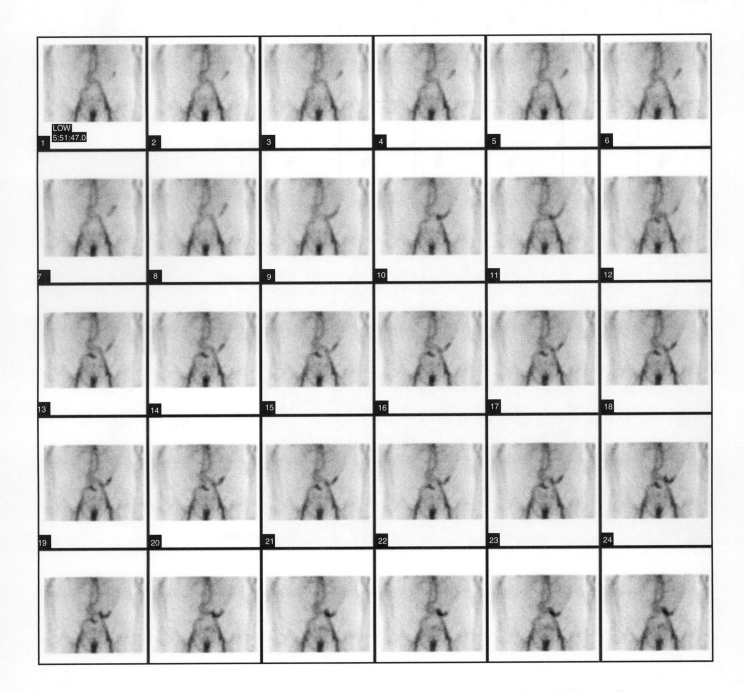

1. What is the pertinent image finding?
   a. Abdominal aortic aneurysm
   b. Ascending colon gastrointestinal bleed
   c. Descending/sigmoid colon gastrointestinal bleed
   d. Descending colon angiodysplasia
2. What is the ideal radiotracer to perform a bleeding scan?
   a. Tc-99m RBC
   b. Tc-99m HMPAO
   c. In-111 white blood cell (WBC)
   d. Tc-99 pertechnetate
3. Which labeling method has the highest efficiency?
   a. In vitro
   b. Modified in vitro
   c. In vivo
   d. Modified in vivo
4. What is the critical organ for a Tc-99m RBC study?
   a. Bladder
   b. Gallbladder
   c. Spleen
   d. Colon

Case 17

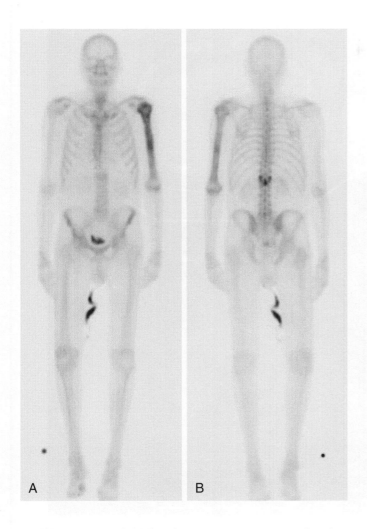

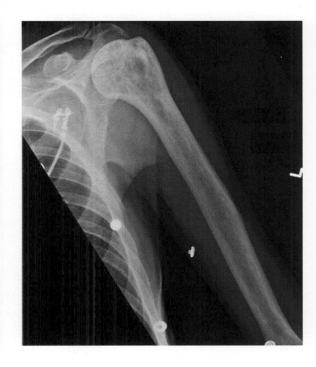

1. This patient with high-risk prostate cancer was referred to rule out metastases. What is your interpretation?
   a. Metastases to humerus and T-12
   b. Metastases to humerus, degenerative disease at T-12
   c. Paget's disease of the humerus and degenerative disease at T-12
   d. Paget's disease of humerus and T-12
2. On radiographs, the affected bone in this disease is likely to have what radiographic appearance?
   a. Coarsened trabeculae and expanded bone
   b. Gracile bones
   c. Associated callus formation
   d. Stress fractures
3. This entity is most commonly diagnosed in the setting of:
   a. Elevated amylase
   b. Elevated alkaline phosphatase
   c. Elevated creatinine
   d. Elevated lipase
4. These patients may suffer complications related to:
   a. Cardiomyopathy
   b. High-output congestive heart failure
   c. Myocarditis
   d. Pericardial effusion

Case 18

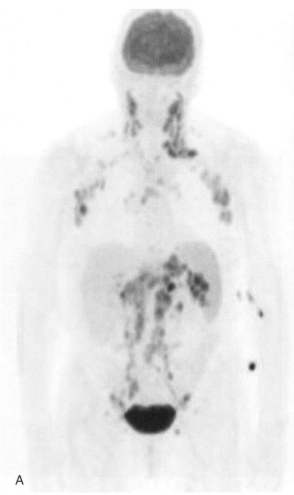

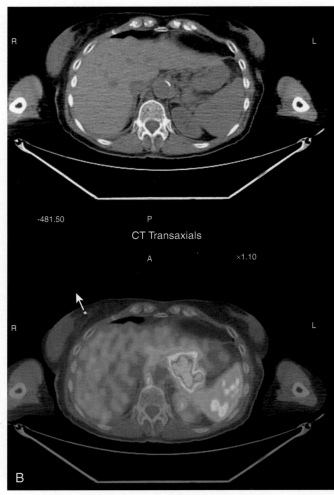

1. F-18 FDG PET/CT scan in a patient with suspected non-Hodgkin's lymphoma (NHL). Other differential considerations include all of the following EXCEPT:
   a. Multicentric Castleman's disease
   b. Metastatic lymphadenopathy
   c. Tuberculosis
   d. Brown fat

2. What stage would this patient with NHL be at according to the Ann Arbor staging system?
   a. Ib
   b. IIa
   c. IIb
   d. III

3. What is a Lugano score?
   a. Assessment of treatment response based on a five-point scale
   b. Assessment of treatment response based on change in absolute standardized uptake value (SUV) values
   c. Maximum standardized uptake value in a voxel
   d. Assessment of treatment response relative to injected FDG dose

4. A Lugano score of 2 is best described as:
   a. Activity above that of liver
   b. Activity similar to that of liver
   c. Activity similar to blood pool
   d. No FDG activity

Case 19

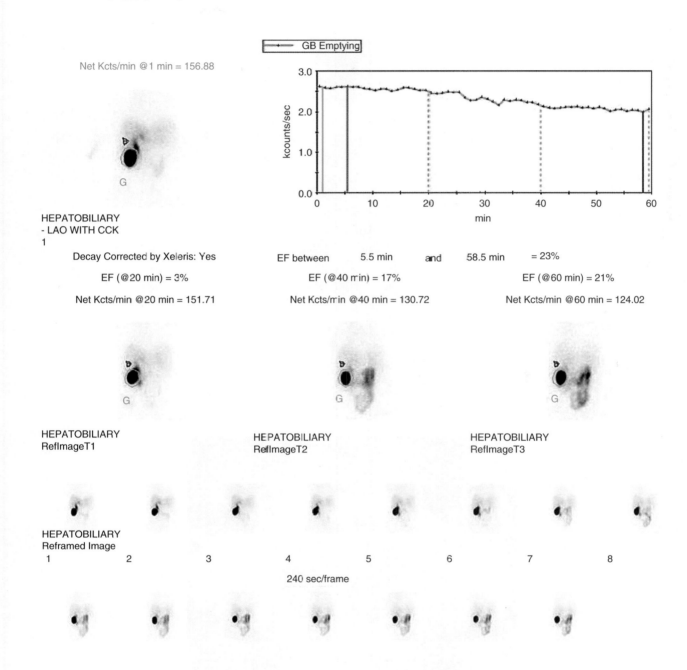

Net Kcts/min @1 min = 156.88

GB Emptying

HEPATOBILIARY
- LAO WITH CCK
1

Decay Corrected by Xeleris: Yes

EF (@20 min) = 3%

Net Kcts/min @20 min = 151.71

EF between   5.5 min   and   58.5 min   = 23%

EF (@40 min) = 17%

Net Kcts/min @40 min = 130.72

EF (@60 min) = 21%

Net Kcts/min @60 min = 124.02

HEPATOBILIARY
RefImageT1

HEPATOBILIARY
RefImageT2

HEPATOBILIARY
RefImageT3

HEPATOBILIARY
Reframed Image
1   2   3   4   5   6   7   8

240 sec/frame

1. What is the salient finding?
   a. Cystic duct obstruction
   b. Abnormal gallbladder contraction
   c. Focal liver lesion
   d. Bile leak
2. What pharmaceutical is infused to evaluate gallbladder contraction?
   a. Cholecystokinin analogue infused as a bolus
   b. Cholecystokinin analogue infused over 60 minutes
   c. Morphine infused as a bolus
   d. Morphine infused over 45 to 60 minutes

3. The lower range of normal for gallbladder ejection fraction is approximately:
   a. 20%
   b. 40%
   c. 60%
   d. 80%
4. What is the possible complication of infusing a cholecystokinin analogue as a bolus?
   a. None reported
   b. Diarrhea
   c. Abdominal cramping
   d. Pancreatitis

Case 20

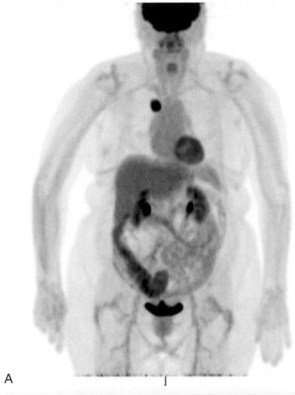

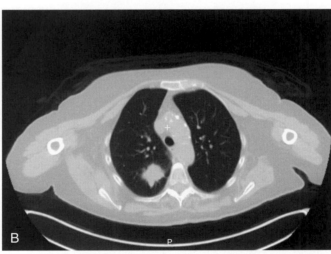

1. What is the most likely diagnosis?
   a. Lung cancer
   b. Esophageal cancer
   c. Lung metastases
   d. Well-differentiated lung carcinoid
2. What is the size criteria for characterizing this lesion as a nodule versus a mass?
   a. A nodule is 3 cm or less in size
   b. A nodule is 2 cm or less in size
   c. A mass is 2 cm or greater in size
   d. No size criteria

3. What is the stage of this patient with primary lung cancer measuring 3 cm in diameter?
   a. Ia
   b. IIb
   c. IIIa
   d. IIIb
4. At which stage is the patient thought to be unresectable at presentation?
   a. I
   b. II
   c. IIIa
   d. IIIb

Case 21

1. What is this QC image?
   a. Four-quadrant bar image
   b. Flood image
   c. Off-peak bone scan image
   d. Thyroid scan
2. Why is this image acquired?
   a. To assess uniformity
   b. To assess linearity
   c. To assess spatial resolution
   d. For attenuation correction
3. How often should this image be acquired?
   a. Daily
   b. Weekly
   c. Monthly
   d. Annually
4. What is the photopeak of cobalt-57 (Co-57) used for this acquisition?
   a. 81 keV
   b. 122 keV
   c. 140 keV
   d. 511 keV

Case 22

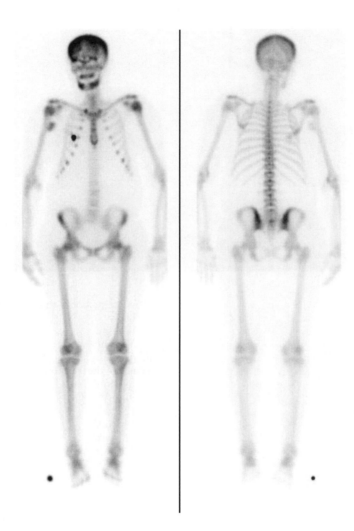

1. What is the salient finding on this bone scan?
   a. Increased uptake in the ribs
   b. Increased uptake in the pelvis
   c. Uptake in the right axilla
   d. Absence of renal uptake
2. What is the most likely explanation for the appearance of this bone scan?
   a. Recent granulocyte colony-stimulating factor (GCSF) therapy
   b. Renal failure
   c. Diffuse metastatic disease
   d. Paget's disease

3. What is a common clinical laboratory finding in renal failure caused by secondary hyperparathyroidism?
   a. Hypocalcemia
   b. Hypercalcemia
   c. Hypophosphatemia
   d. Hypokalemia
4. What is the optimal imaging time after injection of the bone radiopharmaceutical?
   a. 1 hour
   b. 3 hours
   c. 6 hours
   d. 24 hours

Case 23

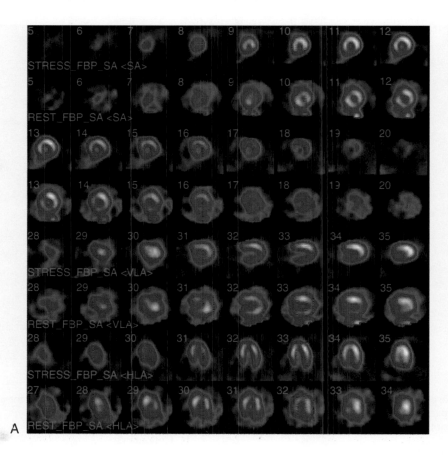

A

1. What is the interpretation of this exercise myocardial perfusion study (Image A)?
   a. Myocardial ischemia
   b. Myocardial infarction
   c. Hibernating myocardium
   d. Normal perfusion
2. Which coronary artery is likely affected?
   a. Left anterior descending
   b. Left circumflex
   c. Left main
   d. Right coronary
3. What determines whether or not a patient should receive an exercise or pharmacologic stress test?
   a. Patient preference
   b. If patient is unable to perform exercise, pharmacologic stress is used
   c. Depends on the clinical diagnosis (i.e., valvular versus coronary artery disease)
   d. Choice of the nuclear physician

4. What is the mechanism of action of regadenoson?
   a. Vasodilation
   b. Vasoconstriction
   c. Ionotropism
   d. Chronotropism

Case 24

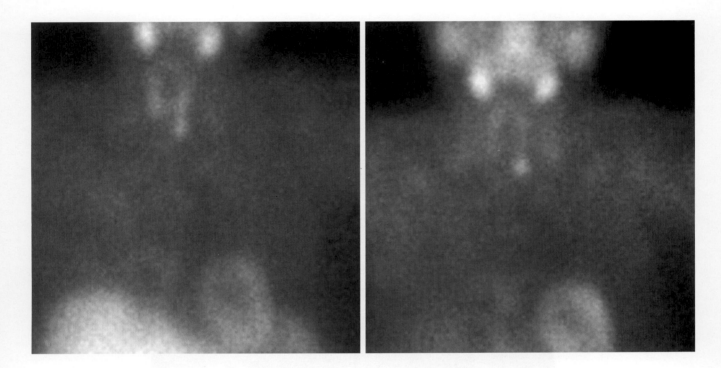

1. What is the purpose of performing a parathyroid study?
   a. Diagnosis of hyperparathyroidism
   b. Exclude hyperparathyroidism in patient with hypercalcemia
   c. Delineate the thyroid gland
   d. Localize the adenoma for surgical planning
2. What is the most common clinical presentation in patients with hyperparathyroidism?
   a. Renal stone
   b. No symptoms
   c. Brown tumors
   d. Fracture
3. What is the most likely etiology for a false-positive result in a parathyroid scintigraphic study?
   a. Thyroid adenoma
   b. Colloid cyst
   c. Lymph nodes
   d. Medullary thyroid cancer
4. Where does the Tc-99m sestamibi localize in a parathyroid adenoma?
   a. Nucleus
   b. Cell membrane
   c. Cytosol
   d. Mitochondria

Case 25

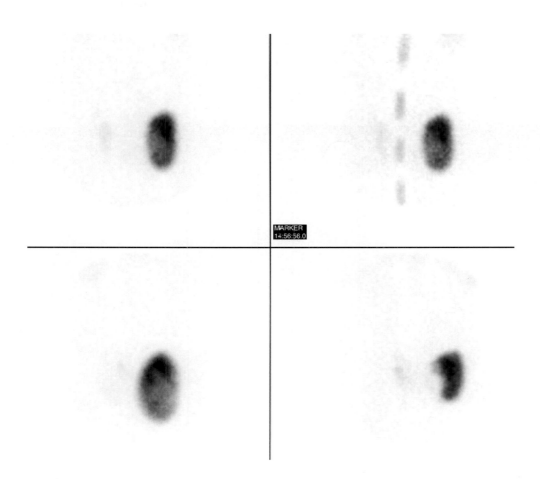

MARKER
14:56:56.0

1. What is the most likely diagnosis in a patient with a suppressed thyroid-stimulating hormone (TSH)?
   a. Subacute thyroiditis
   b. Multinodular goiter
   c. Autonomous toxic nodule
   d. Papillary thyroid cancer
2. What is the most likely 24-hour uptake value?
   a. Less than 1%
   b. 20%
   c. 50%
   d. Greater than 80%

3. What is the most likely treatment choice?
   a. Radiation
   b. I-131 therapy
   c. Tyrosine kinase inhibitors
   d. Synthroid
4. If I-131 therapy is administered, what is the most likely dose?
   a. 10 mCi
   b. 25 mCi
   c. 50 mCi
   d. 100 mCi

Case 26

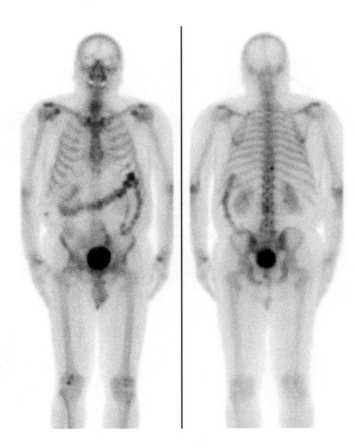

1. What is the most likely cause for the colon uptake on this bone scan in a patient with no clinical symptoms or complaints?
   a. Radiolabeling error
   b. Metformin therapy
   c. Diverticulitis
   d. Recent scintigraphic study
2. What scintigraphic study is most likely to be responsible?
   a. In-111 leukocyte study
   b. Tc-99m myocardial perfusion study
   c. Tc-99m DSMA
   d. Tc-99m RBC scan
3. What is the explanation for this finding?
   a. The Tc-99m cardiac radiotracer is excreted by liver into bowel
   b. Erroneous oral ingestion of radiotracer rather than intravenous injection
   c. Wrong radiotracer administered
   d. Renal dysfunction
4. What is the role of the stannous ion in the methyl diphosphonate (MDP) kit formulation?
   a. Bind and remove alumina contamination
   b. Prevent breakdown of radiopharmaceutical over time
   c. Acts as a reducing agent to facilitate binding of the Tc-99m to the MDP molecule
   d. Sterilize the preparation

Case 27

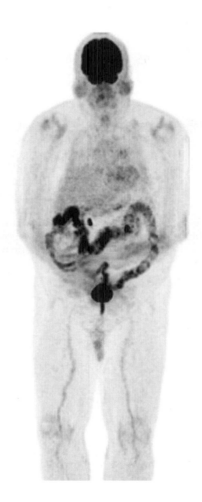

1. The patient is likely being treated for what condition?
   a. Diabetes mellitus
   b. Graves' disease
   c. Hypertension
   d. Hyperlipidemia
2. The patient is most likely taking what medication?
   a. Insulin
   b. Propranolol
   c. Valium
   d. Metformin
3. The high brain F-18 FDG uptake is caused by:
   a. Cerebritis
   b. Normal physiology

c. The same reason as for intestinal uptake
d. Patient being mentally alert (watching TV during uptake time)

4. How should the patient be instructed to prepare for an F-18 FDG PET/CT scan?
   a. Nothing per mouth (NPO) for 4 to 6 hours and no long-acting insulin for 12 hours before scanning
   b. No need to be NPO and no change in insulin administration
   c. NPO for 12 to 24 hours and may take long-acting insulin the morning of examination
   d. No need to be NPO and no long-acting insulin the morning of the examination

Case 28

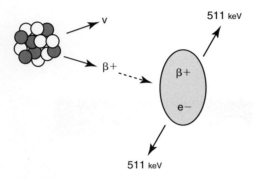

2. An alpha particle consists of:
   a. One proton and one neutron
   b. Two protons and one neutron
   c. Two protons and two neutrons
   d. One proton and two neutrons
3. For positron decay to occur, the transition energy must be in excess of:
   a. 511 keV
   b. 711 keV
   c. 1022 keV
   d. 1422 keV
4. What is the process called when two 511-keV photons are produced for PET imaging?
   a. Incidence detection
   b. Annihilation
   c. Internal conversion
   d. Isomeric transition

1. All of the following are modes of radioactive decay of radio-nuclides utilized in the nuclear medicine clinic EXCEPT:
   a. Electron capture
   b. Beta
   c. Positron
   d. Epsilon

Case 29

Initial Imaging

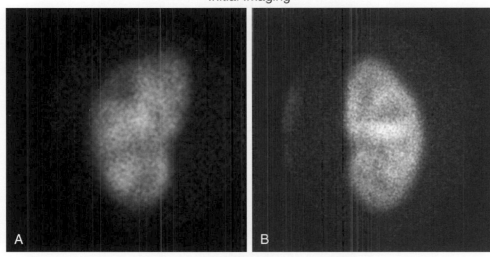

Follow up Imaging

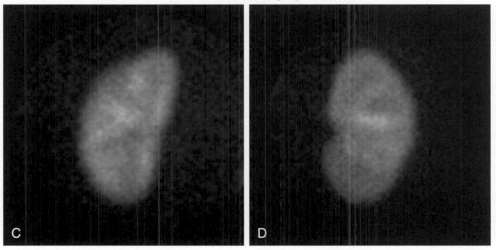

1. Interpret the Tc-99m DMSA planar images:
   a. Renal scars
   b. Acute pyelonephritis
   c. Reflux
   d. Tumor
2. What is the primary mechanism of Tc-99m DMSA uptake?
   a. Is secreted through the distal tubules
   b. Is secreted through the proximal tubules
   c. Binds to the proximal renal tubules
   d. Binds to the loop of Henle
3. Indications for Tc-99m DMSA imaging include all EXCEPT:
   a. Obstruction
   b. Split renal function
   c. Cortical scarring
   d. Pyelonephritis
4. The most common cause of pyelonephritis is:
   a. Obstruction
   b. Reflux disease
   c. Renal mass
   d. Systemic infection

Case 30

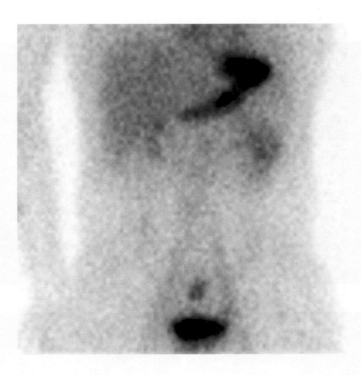

1. What is the radiotracer used for a Meckel's diverticulum study?
   a. Tc-99m sulfur colloid
   b. Tc-99m DSMA
   c. Tc-99m RBC
   d. Tc 99m pertechnetate
2. What pharmacologic agent is often used to improve detection of this entity?
   a. Cimetidine
   b. Valium
   c. Potassium perchlorate
   d. Pentagastrin
3. What is the most common cause for a false-positive result?
   a. Activity within the gastrointestinal (GI) tract
   b. Activity within the urinary tract
   c. Inflammatory bowel disease
   d. Enteric duplication cyst
4. What is the incidence of Meckel's diverticulum in children?
   a. 2%
   b. 10%
   c. 20%
   d. 22%

Case 31

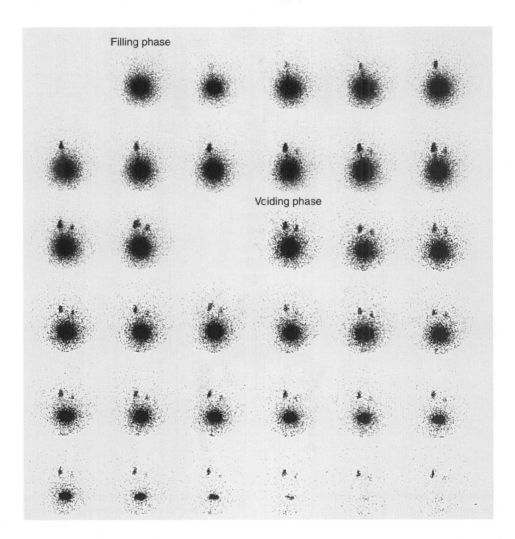

Filling phase

Vciding phase

1. What is the likely radiopharmaceutical?
   a. Tc-99m MAG3
   b. Tc-99m pertechnetate
   c. Tc-99m DMSA
   d. Tc-99m DTPA
2. What is the diagnosis?
   a. Urinary reflux
   b. Pyelonephritis
   c. Wilms' tumor
   d. Ureterocele

3. How would you grade the activity on the left?
   a. I
   b. II
   c. III
   d. IV
4. What is the advantage of radionuclide cystography over voiding cystourethrography?
   a. None
   b. Lower radiation dose
   c. Decreased sensitivity for detection of reflux
   d. Increased anatomic information

Case 32

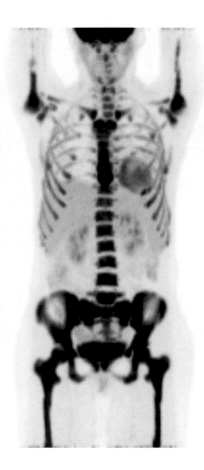

1. What is the most likely etiology for these findings?
   a. Recent chemotherapy and GCSF administration
   b. Recent physical activity
   c. Failure to fast before scanning
   d. Trauma
2. What is the ideal time of F-18 FDG PET/CT imaging in patients receiving marrow-stimulating therapies?
   a. On the first day of therapy
   b. Any time during therapy
   c. After the effects of therapy have resolved
   d. Day after final administration
3. Increased bone marrow uptake may result in:
   a. Increased risk of marrow-related tumor
   b. Masking of true neoplastic osseous lesions
   c. Increased risk of fracture
   d. Nondiagnostic scan
4. What is the purpose of adding GCSF to a patient's regimen?
   a. To treat myelosuppression induced by chemotherapy
   b. Increase detection of lesions on FDG PET/CT
   c. Enhance chemotherapy effect
   d. Reduced inflammation related to chemotherapy

Case 33

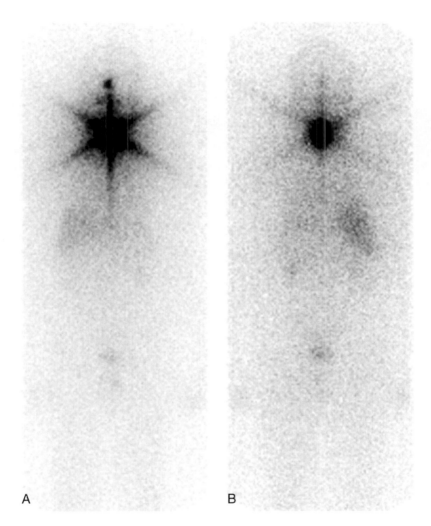

A   B

1. What is the radionuclide?
   a. I-123
   b. I-131
   c. I-124
   d. Tc-99m
2. What is this uptake pattern called?
   a. Star artifact
   b. Moon artifact
   c. Pinhole artifact
   d. Ring artifact

3. What causes this finding?
   a. Collimator septa breakdown
   b. Penetration of collimator septa by high-energy photons
   c. Increased width of the crystal
   d. Injection site in the field of view
4. What is the probable cause for liver uptake in this patient?
   a. Thyroid hormone metabolism
   b. Metastases
   c. Misadministration
   d. Fatty liver disease

Case 34

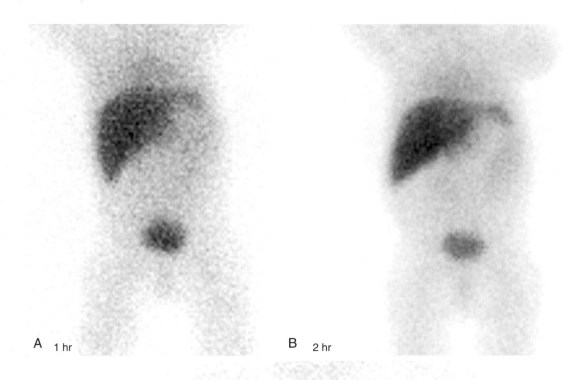

A 1 hr

B 2 hr

C 24 hr

1. What is the radiopharmaceutical?
   a. Tc-99m mebrofenin
   b. Tc-99m RBC
   c. Tc-99m pertechnetate
   d. Tc-99m HMPAO
2. What is the best diagnosis in this neonate?
   a. Findings consistent with biliary atresia
   b. No evidence of biliary atresia
   c. Neonatal hepatitis
   d. Biliary atresia versus neonatal hepatitis

3. What is the recommended preparation for this test?
   a. NPO only
   b. Phenobarbital for 5 days before examination
   c. Phenobarbital the day of examination
   d. Cimetidine 2 days before examination
4. This study has: (*Select the best answer.*)
   a. High sensitivity
   b. High specificity
   c. Low sensitivity
   d. Low specificity

Case 35

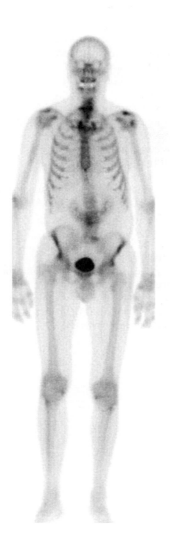

1. What is the most important finding on this bone scan?
   a. Abnormal thyroid uptake
   b. Degenerative disease
   c. Renal anomaly
   d. Adrenal uptake
2. What is the most likely diagnosis?
   a. Horseshoe kidney
   b. Renal cancer
   c. Adrenal hyperplasia
   d. Intra-abdominal malignancy
3. Patients who have a horseshoe kidney are at increased risk for:
   a. Veno-occlusive disease
   b. Renal stones
   c. Lymphatic obstruction
   d. Breast cancer
4. Peak bone radiotracer uptake occurs at:
   a. 1 hour
   b. 2 hours
   c. 3 hours
   d. 4 hours

Case 36

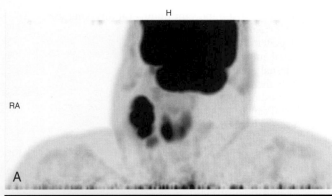

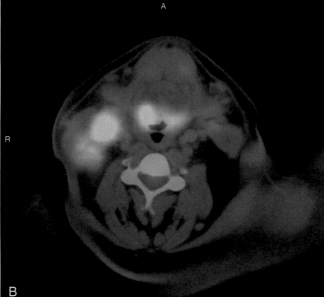

1. What is the most likely diagnosis on this F-18 FDG PET/CT in a patient who has had no intervention?
   a. Thyroid carcinoma
   b. Cervical paraganglioma
   c. Warthin's tumors
   d. Head and neck carcinoma
2. The most common histology for head and neck cancers is:
   a. Adenocarcinoma
   b. Squamous cell carcinoma
   c. Round cell tumor
   d. Small cell carcinoma
3. A synchronous second primary malignancy is most likely to be found in:
   a. Lungs
   b. Colon
   c. Kidneys
   d. Reproductive organs
4. The presence of head and neck cancer may be associated with:
   a. Herpes virus
   b. Cytomegalovirus (CMV)
   c. Human papilloma virus (HPV)
   d. Respiratory syncytial virus (RSV)

Case 37

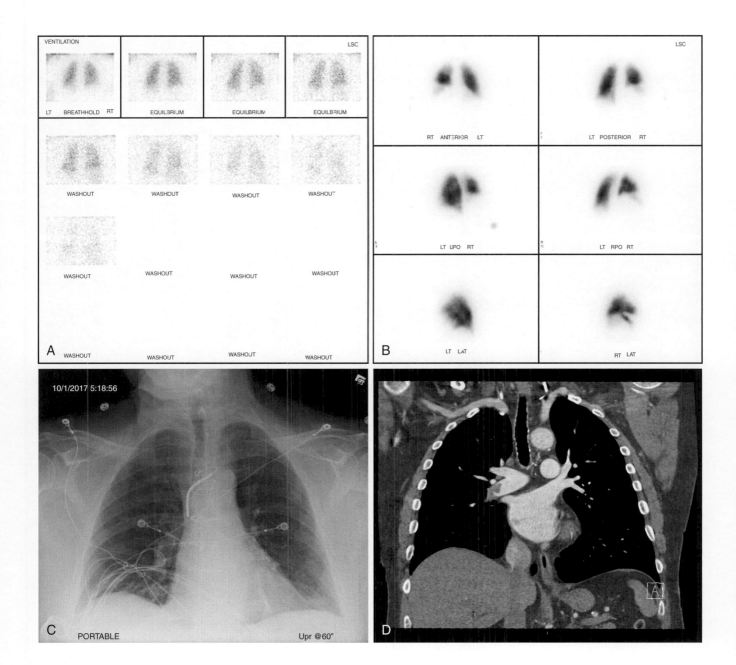

1. How would you interpret this lung scan in a patient with acute shortness of breath and a normal result on chest radiography?
   a. Normal
   b. Low probability of pulmonary embolism (PE)
   c. Intermediate probability of PE
   d. High probability of PE
2. What is the probability of PE in this patient?
   a. Less than 5%
   b. Less than 20%
   c. Approximately 33%
   d. Greater than 80%

3. What is the radiopharmaceutical used for perfusion?
   a. Xenon-133 (Xe-133)
   b. Tc-99 DTPA
   c. Tc-99 MAA
   d. Tc-99 DSMA
4. What is the radiopharmaceutical used for ventilation in this study?
   a. Xe-133
   b. Tc-99 DTPA
   c. Tc-99 MAA
   d. Tc-99 DSMA

Case 38

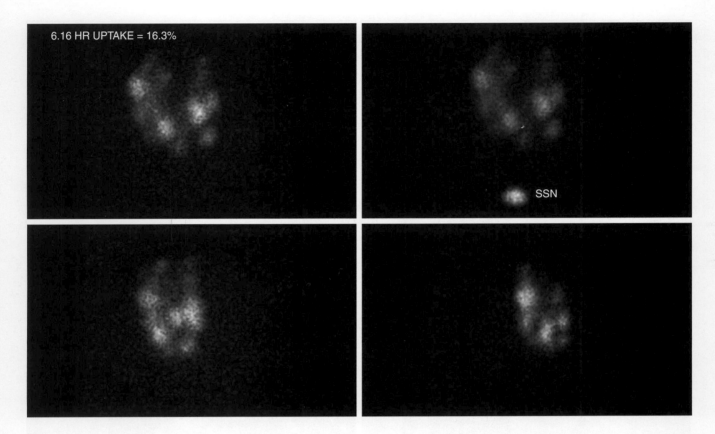

1. What is the diagnosis in a patient with low TSH?
   a. Graves' disease
   b. Subacute thyroiditis
   c. Multinodular toxic goiter
   d. Papillary thyroid cancer
2. What is the likelihood of thyroid cancer in this patient?
   a. 30%
   b. 20%
   c. 15%
   d. Less than 5%

3. If this patient were to be treated with I-131, what would be the most likely dose?
   a. 10 mCi
   b. 15 mCi
   c. 25 mCi
   d. 50 mCi
4. What is the half-life of I-123?
   a. 2.8 hours
   b. 13 hours
   c. 6 hours
   d. 8 days

Case 39

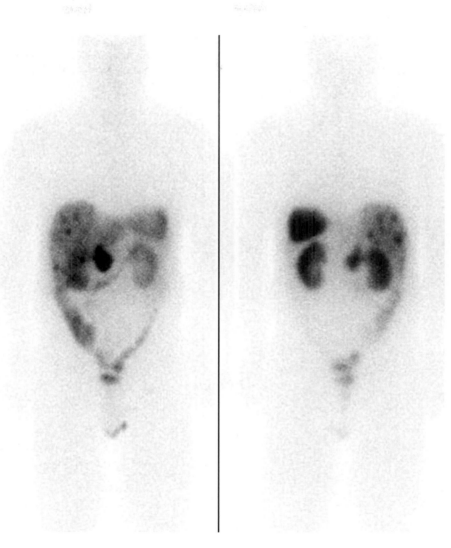

1. In-111 OctreoScan has highest sensitivity for:
   a. Insulinoma
   b. Meningioma
   c. Carcinoid
   d. Medullary thyroid cancer
2. The half-life of Indium-111 is:
   a. 6 hours
   b. 13 hours
   c. 67 hours
   d. 78 hours

3. OctreoScan has low sensitivity for detection of which of the following:
   a. Carcinoid tumor
   b. Adrenomedullary tumor
   c. Insulinoma
   d. Gastrinoma
4. An alternative somatostatin imaging radiopharmaceutical is:
   a. Ga-68 DOTATATE PET/CT
   b. Amyloid PET/CT
   c. Sodium flucride (NaF) PET/CT
   d. F-18 DOPA PET/CT

Case 40

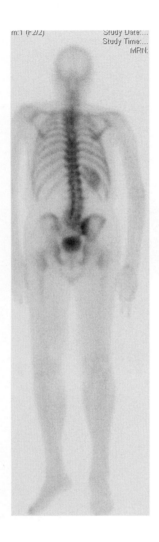

1. What is the salient finding?
   a. Radiotracer-avid lesion in the right sacroiliac region
   b. Photopenic lesion in the left sacroiliac region
   c. Right lower rib lesion
   d. Absent right kidney
2. What is the most likely diagnosis?
   a. Renal cell cancer
   b. Lymphoma
   c. Multiple myeloma
   d. Breast cancer
3. A focal photopenic osseous defect on this bone scan is most likely to represent:
   a. Bone cyst
   b. Metastasis
   c. Contamination of urine
   d. Degenerative changes
4. What is the photopeak window set by the technologist when acquiring this image?
   a. 126–154 keV
   b. 100–140 keV
   c. 140–165 keV
   d. 13–141 keV

Case 41

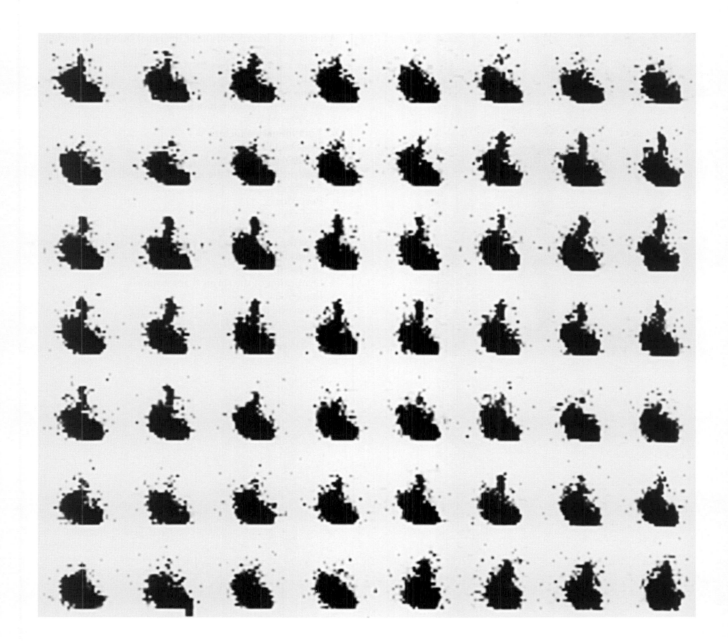

1. The primary purpose of this study is to detect:
   a. Pulmonary aspiration
   b. Gastroesophageal reflux
   c. Esophageal transit rate
   d. Gastric emptying
2. What is the optimal acquisition framing rate?
   a. 5–10 seconds/frame
   b. 1 minute/frame
   c. 5 minutes/frame
   d. 10 minutes/frame

3. What is the most sensitive scintigraphic method for evaluation of aspiration?
   a. Milk study
   b. Salivagraphy
   c. Liquid gastric emptying study
   d. Solid gastric emptying study
4. In what group of patients is this study most commonly performed?
   a. 40- to 60-year-olds
   b. 20- to 40-year-olds
   c. 10- to 20-year-olds
   d. Infants

Case 42

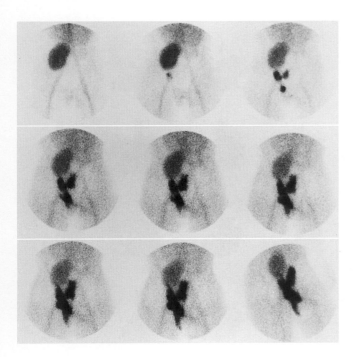

1. What is your interpretation of the renal transplant study?
   a. Obstruction
   b. Acute tubular necrosis
   c. Leak
   d. Acute rejection
2. What is the preferred radiotracer?
   a. Tc-99m MAG3
   b. Tc-99m pertechnetate
   c. Tc-99m DTPA
   d. Tc-99m DMSA
3. In what projection are the images acquired?
   a. Anterior
   b. Posterior
   c. Right lateral
   d. Right anterior oblique
4. What is the most likely cause for this finding in the perioperative period?
   a. Infection
   b. Disruption of the surgical anastomosis
   c. Rejection
   d. Cadaveric donor

Case 43

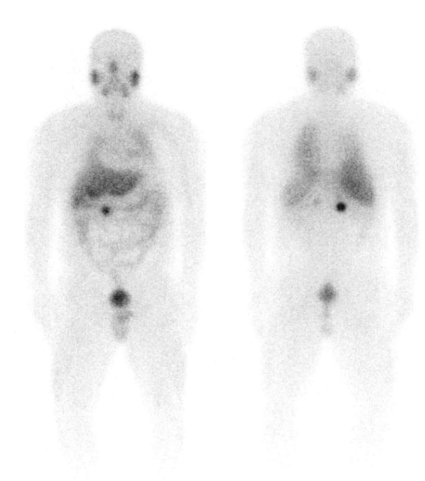

A   B

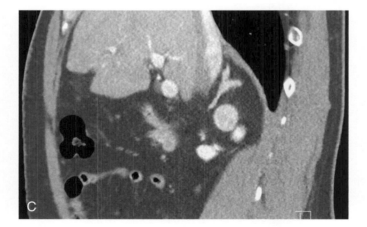

1. The radiopharmaceutical used for this study resembles what hormone?
   a. Norepinephrine
   b. Epinephrine
   c. Vasopressin
   d. Dopamine

2. What is your interpretation of the study?
   a. Paraganglioma
   b. Adrenal cortical carcinoma
   c. Pheochromocytoma
   d. Metastatic disease

3. This radiotracer is useful for the diagnosis of what other disease?
   a. Lymphoma
   b. Neuroblastoma
   c. Thyroid cancer
   d. Adrenal medullary hyperplasia

4. Which drug can interfere with the uptake of the radiopharmaceutical?
   a. Valium
   b. Labetalol
   c. Histamine 2 (H_2) receptor antagonists
   d. Dramamine

Case 44

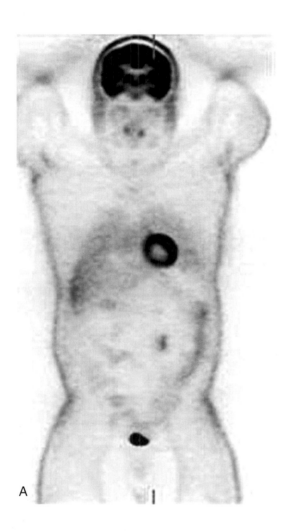

A

B

1. How would you characterize these images?
   a. Non–attenuation-corrected (NAC) PET images
   b. NAC and attenuation-corrected (AC) images
   c. Subtraction PET images
   d. AC images
2. Attenuation correction can be performed with all of the following EXCEPT:
   a. CT
   b. Germanium-68 rod
   c. Cesium-137 rod
   d. Technetium rod
3. What lesions may be best seen on NAC images?
   a. Skin
   b. Kidney
   c. Heart
   d. Pancreas

4. The NAC images should be inspected in all the following scenarios EXCEPT:
   a. Increased uptake in the region of surgical clips
   b. Focal uptake in the pancreatic head
   c. Liver lesion activity misregistered because of diaphragmatic excursion
   d. Lung lesion activity misregistered because of patient's breathing

Case 45

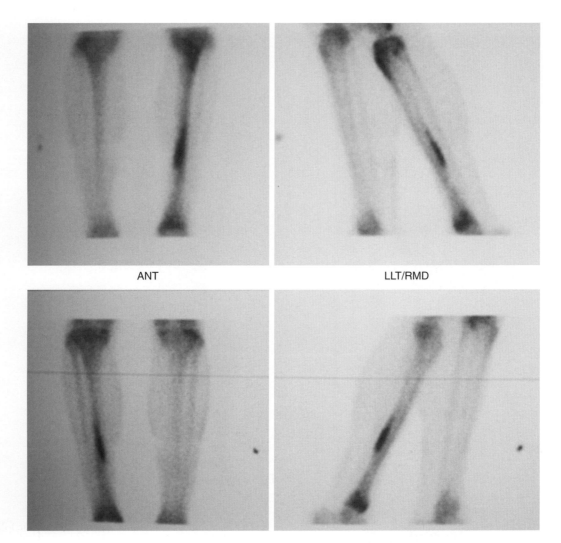

ANT   LLT/RMD

1. What is the salient finding?
   a. Increased radiotracer uptake along the posteromedial aspect of the left tibia consistent with a fracture
   b. Increased radiotracer uptake along the posteromedial aspect of the left tibia consistent with shin splints
   c. Increased radiotracer uptake along the posteromedial aspect of the left tibia consistent with metastases
   d. Increased radiotracer uptake along the posteromedial aspect of the left tibia consistent with normal physiologic activity
2. What is the most common finding on three-phase bone scintigraphy of a stress fracture?
   a. Flow, blood pool, and delayed imaging positive with diffuse bony uptake on delayed imaging
   b. Flow and blood pool negative, focal cortical uptake on delayed imaging
   c. Flow and blood pool negative, diffuse bony uptake on delayed imaging
   d. Flow, blood pool, and delayed imaging positive with focal cortical uptake on delayed imaging
3. Most fractures become detectable on bone scintigraphy after:
   a. 1 day
   b. 5 days
   c. 1 week
   d. 1 month
4. What is the most likely etiology in this case?
   a. Acute trauma
   b. Repetitive trauma resulting in periostitis at the insertion sites of the tibialis and soleus muscles
   c. Medication-induced alteration in bone turnover
   d. Repetitive trauma resulting in periostitis at the insertion sites of the hamstring muscles

Case 46

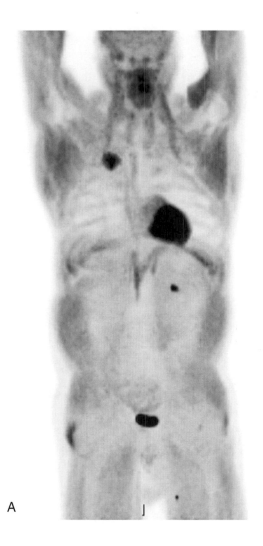

A

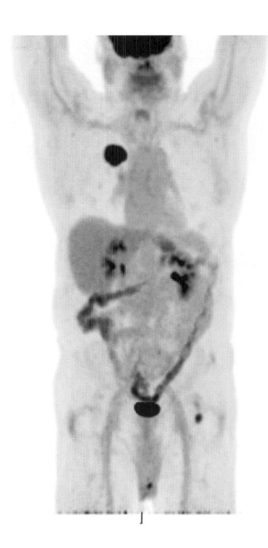

B

1. What is the explanation for the abnormal uptake distribution on the F-18 FDG PET study? (See Image A.)
   a. Patient ate shortly before injection
   b. Wrong radiopharmaceutical
   c. Recent physical exercise
   d. Too short a time interval from injection to imaging
2. FDG is a:
   a. Glucose analogue
   b. Fructose analogue
   c. Methionine analogue
   d. Hydroxyapatite analogue
3. How long are patients required to fast before the study?
   a. 2 hours
   b. 4 hours
   c. 8 hours
   d. 12 hours
4. The usual imaging delay between injection and scan time for F-18 FDG PET/CT usually is:
   a. 30 minutes
   b. 60 minutes
   c. 90 minutes
   d. 120 minutes

Case 47

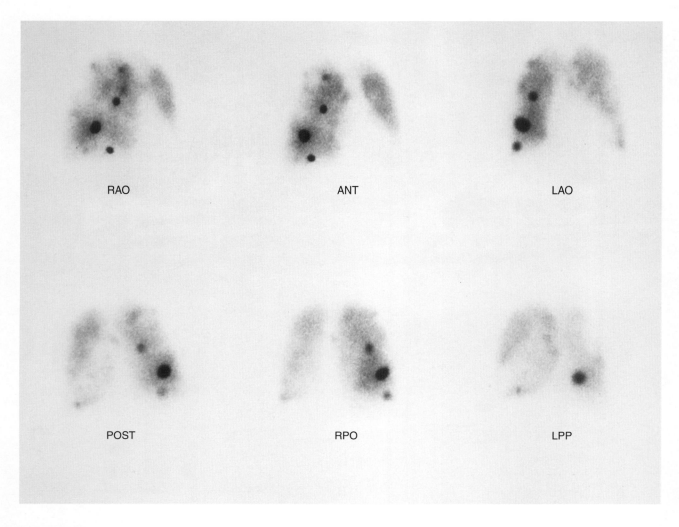

RAO ANT LAO

POST RPO LPP

1. What is the most likely etiology for the imaging finding?
   a. Metastases
   b. Pulmonary emboli
   c. Technical
   d. Multiple arteriovenous malformations (AVMs)
2. What is the likely cause for this finding?
   a. Wrong radiopharmaceutical injected
   b. Wrong photopeak selected by the technologist
   c. Blood in the syringe before injection
   d. Incomplete ventilation study

3. What is the perfusion agent for the study?
   a. Tc-99m MAA
   b. Xe-133
   c. Tc-99m DTPA
   d. Technegas
4. If the patient has pulmonary hypertension, what would you consider altering in the protocol?
   a. Eliminating the ventilation images
   b. Eliminating the perfusion images
   c. Increasing the number of MAA particles
   d. Reducing the number of MAA particles

Case 48

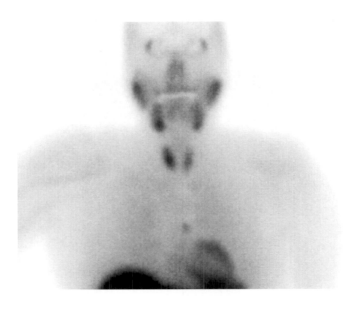

1. All of the following scans may demonstrate normal physiologic distribution of tracer to the thyroid EXCEPT:
   a. Iodine-123 (I-123) metaiodobenzylguanidine (MIBG)
   b. Technetium-99m (Tc-99m) sestamibi
   c. Indium-111 (In-111) oxine white blood cell (WBC)
   d. Tc-99m pertechnetate
2. Which scan is shown?
   a. Tc-99m pertechnetate
   b. Tc-99m sestamibi
   c. In-111 WBC
   d. In-111 pentetreotide

3. Where is the abnormal uptake?
   a. Right thyroid lobe
   b. Lacrimal glands
   c. Parotid glands
   d. Mediastinum
4. A patient presents with elevated serum calcium, decreased serum phosphorus, and elevated parathyroid hormone. What is the referring physician evaluating for?
   a. Toxic thyroid nodule
   b. Parathyroid adenoma
   c. Medullary thyroid carcinoma
   d. Graves' disease

Case 49

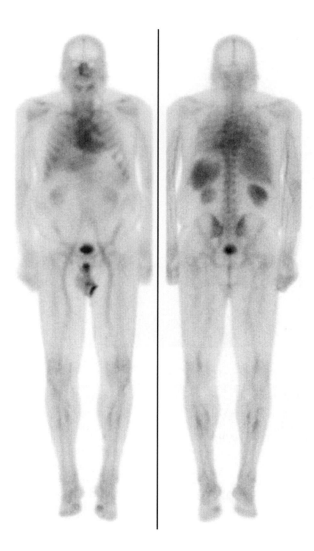

1. A scan was acquired approximately 3 hours after injection. What radiopharmaceutical has been given for this study?
   a. Tc-99m sestamibi
   b. Tc-99m methyl diphosphonate (MDP)
   c. Tc-99m red blood cell (RBC)
   d. In-111 oxine WBC
2. There is unexpected extraosseous activity in all of the following EXCEPT:
   a. Heart
   b. Urinary bladder
   c. Spleen
   d. Liver
3. Differential considerations for extraosseous activity on a bone scan include:
   a. Metastatic disease
   b. Oxidation and breakdown of the radiolabeled compound with release of free pertechnetate
   c. Residual activity from a previous radionuclide procedure
   d. All of the above
4. Further inquiry into the patient's clinical history reveals that he is being treated with doxorubicin for his urinary bladder cancer. He says that he had a recent test in the Nuclear Medicine department. Which of the following tests would account for the extraosseous activity?
   a. Tc-99m sestamibi myocardial perfusion scan
   b. In-111 WBC scan
   c. Fluorine-18 (F-18) PET scan
   d. Multigated acquisition (MUGA) cardiac blood scan

Case 50

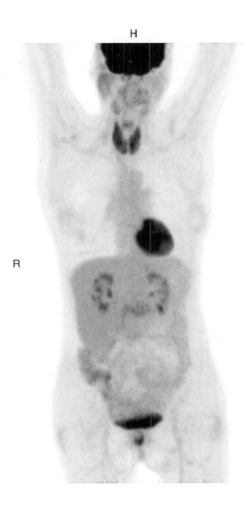

H

R

1. Fluorodeoxyglucose (FDG) positron emission tomography (PET) is requested for a patient referred for restaging of previously treated breast cancer. There is no history of thyroid disease. Statistically, what is the most likely diagnosis for the diffuse uptake in the thyroid?
   a. Medullary thyroid cancer
   b. Papillary thyroid carcinoma
   c. Graves' disease
   d. Chronic lymphocytic thyroiditis
2. Further standard workup may involve all of the following EXCEPT:
   a. Serum thyroid-stimulating hormone (TSH), free thyroxine
   b. Serum lactate dehydrogenase (LDH)
   c. Thyroid ultrasonography
   d. Antithyroid antibodies

3. Normal thyroid gland appearance on FDG PET can be best characterized as?
   a. No uptake
   b. Mild heterogeneous uptake maximum standardized uptake value (SUV_{max}) less than 2.0
   c. Focal uptake if there a nodule seen on computed tomography (CT)
   d. Heterogeneous uptake with SUV_{max} greater than 2.0
4. How might Hashimoto's thyroiditis be treated in the setting of hypothyroidism?
   a. I-131 (<30 mCi)
   b. I-131 (>30 mCi)
   c. Levothyroxine
   d. Propranolol

Case 51

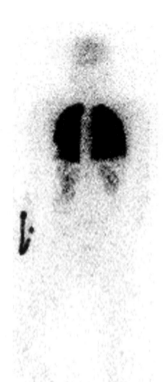

A whole-body posterior planar image from a nuclear medicine study is shown.

1. What is the administered radiopharmaceutical?
   a. Tc-99m hydroxydiphosphonate (HDP)
   b. Tc-99m macroaggregated albumin (MAA)
   c. Xenon-133 (Xe-133)
   d. Tc-99m diethylene-triamine-penta-acetate (DTPA)

2. There is abnormal uptake in what organs?
   a. Brain and lungs
   b. Lungs and kidneys
   c. Brain and kidneys
   d. Brain, kidneys, and lungs

3. All of the following could account for the findings in the scan, EXCEPT:
   a. Eisenmenger's syndrome
   b. Hepatopulmonary syndrome
   c. Ebstein's anomaly
   d. Pulmonary embolism

4. What underlying pathophysiologic process is depicted in the scan?
   a. Left-to-right shunt
   b. Right-to-left shunt
   c. Pulmonary arterial hypertension
   d. Systemic hypertension

Case 52

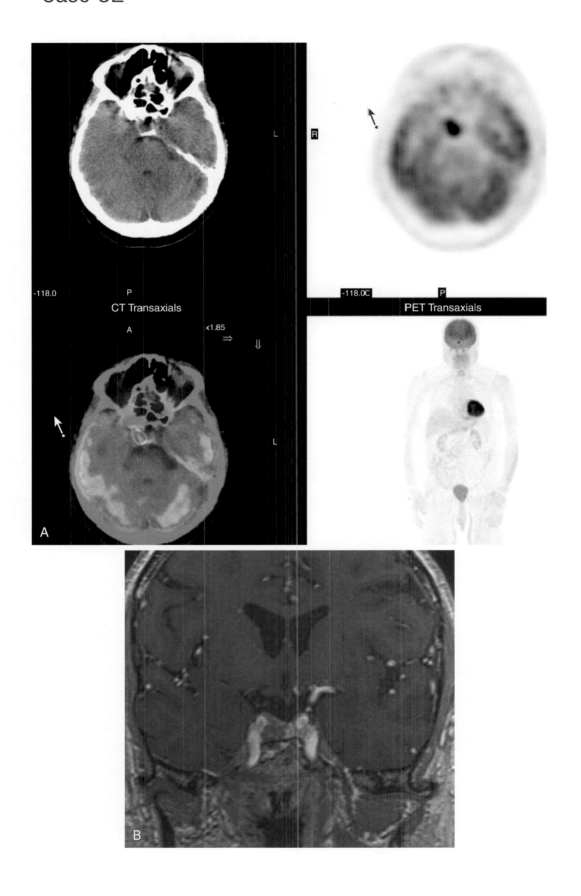

1. Multiple F-18-FDG PET/CT images from a patient being initially evaluated for a single pulmonary nodule are shown. The focal activity on the PET/CT images is most likely localizing to what structure?
   a. Amygdala
   b. Sella turcica
   c. Sphenoid sinus
   d. Optic chiasm

2. On the basis of the FDG PET/CT images alone, all of the following would be included in the differential EXCEPT:
   a. Metastatic disease
   b. Lymphocytic hypophysitis
   c. Pituitary adenoma
   d. Rathke's cleft cyst

3. The patient's FDG PET/CT scan was otherwise negative, and coronal magnetic resonance imaging (MRI) of the brain was ordered after the PET/CT. What is the most likely diagnosis?
   a. Pituitary adenoma
   b. Metastasis
   c. Rathke's cleft cyst
   d. Pituitary hyperplasia

4. What statement best characterizes normal pituitary gland appearance on FDG PET/CT?
   a. Focal photopenia
   b. No to low-level uniform uptake
   c. Low-level uptake in the pituitary stalk
   d. Intense, heterogeneous uptake in the gland, above that of adjacent cerebral cortices

Case 53

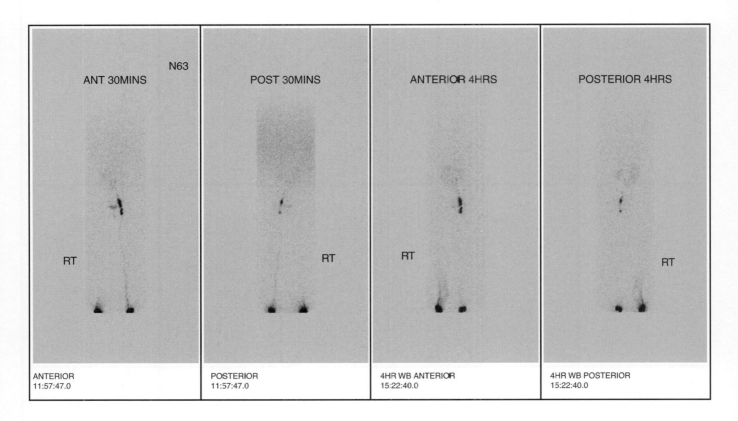

ANT 30MINS

POST 30MINS

ANTERIOR 4HRS

POSTERIOR 4HRS

RT

RT

RT

RT

ANTERIOR
11:57:47.0

POSTERIOR
11:57:47.0

4HR WB ANTERIOR
15:22:40.0

4HR WB POSTERIOR
15:22:40.0

1. A 35-year-old male presents with recurrent right foot and leg swelling and multiple episodes of right leg cellulitis. Anterior and posterior whole-body scintigraphy was performed at 30 minutes and 4 hours. What is the radiopharmaceutical used in the study?
   a. Tc99m pertechnetate
   b. Tc99m SC
   c. Sodium (Na) I-131
   d. Tc-99m MDP
2. Where was the radiopharmaceutical injected?
   a. Interdigital web spaces of the bilateral feet
   b. Interdigital web spaces of the left foot only
   c. Left groin
   d. Right antecubital fossa

3. All of the following are findings on scintigraphy associated with lower extremity lymphedema EXCEPT:
   a. Dermal backflow
   b. Absent or asymmetric visualization of lymph nodes, lymphatic trunks
   c. Presence of lymphatic collateral vessels or dilated lymphatics
   d. Visualization of inguinal lymph nodes
4. What is the salient finding?
   a. Lymphatic obstruction both lower extremities
   b. Lymphatic obstruction right lower extremity
   c. Lymphatic obstruction left lower extremity
   d. Normal study

Case 54

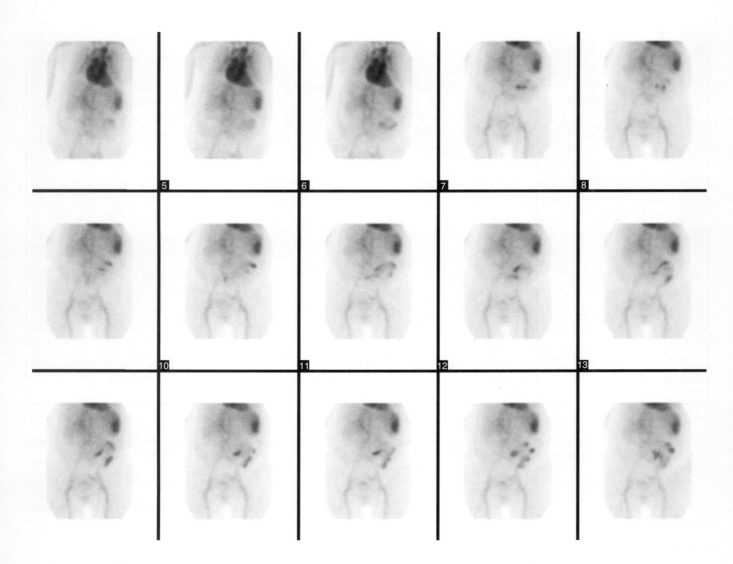

A series of 1-minute images from a Tc-99m–labeled RBC gastrointestinal bleed study are shown.

1. What is the likely diagnosis?
   a. Transverse colon bleed
   b. Jejunal bleed
   c. Rectal bleed
   d. Descending colon bleed
2. If the RBC labeling is not available, what other radiopharmaceutical could be used to detect a GI bleed?
   a. Tc-99m DTPA
   b. Tc-99m pertechnetate
   c. Tc-99m mebrofenin
   d. Tc-99m SC

3. Which of the following statements is true?
   a. Nuclear medicine scintigraphy is 10 times less sensitive than catheter-directed contrast angiography in the detection of GI bleeding
   b. Nuclear medicine scintigraphy is 10 times more sensitive than catheter-directed contrast angiography in the detection of GI bleeding
   c. Nuclear medicine scintigraphy is 100 times more sensitive than catheter-directed contrast angiography in the detection of GI bleeding
   d. Nuclear medicine scintigraphy is similar in sensitivity to that of catheter-directed contrast angiography in the detection of GI bleeding
4. Potential pitfalls in the interpretation of Tc-99m SC scans include all of the following EXCEPT:
   a. Liver uptake
   b. Accessory spleen uptake
   c. Uptake in abdominal varices
   d. All of the above

Case 55

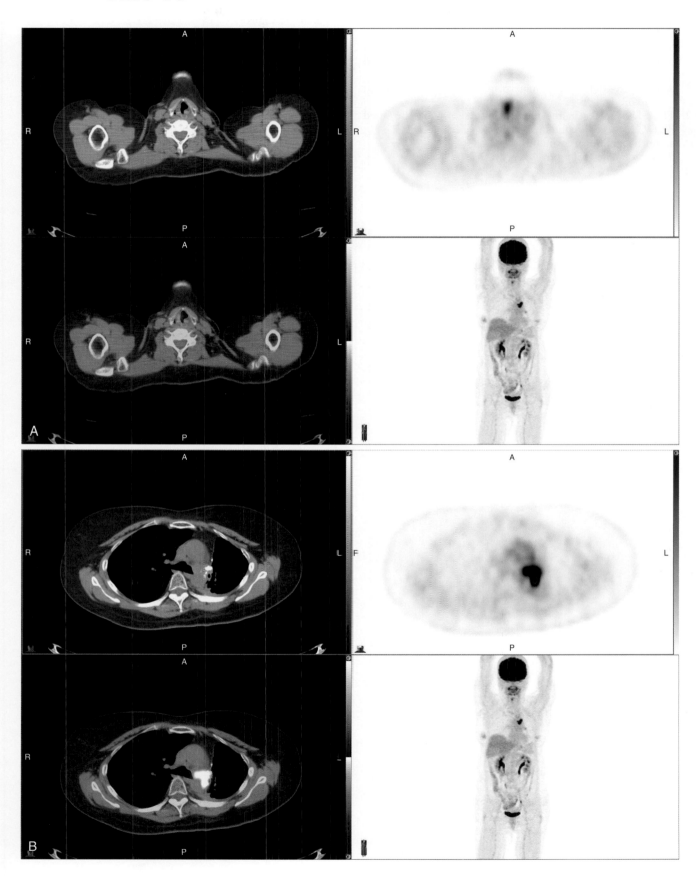

1. A patient who has had a prior left upper lobectomy for lung cancer is referred for PET/CT with new-onset hoarseness. On the fused PET/CT images, at the level of the larynx, the unilateral right-sided vocal cord FDG uptake is caused by which of the following?
   a. Malignant involvement of the right vocal cord
   b. Inflammatory infiltration of the right vocal cord
   c. Compensation by and hypertrophy of the nonparalyzed cord on the right
   d. Compensation by and hypertrophy of the nonparalyzed cord on the left
2. The FDG uptake in the mediastinum shown on the fused PET/CT images is contained in what space?
   a. Aorticopulmonary window
   b. Azygoesophageal groove
   c. Prevascular space
   d. Subcarinal space
3. Which nerve is likely responsible for the vocal cord paralysis in this case?
   a. Right vagus
   b. Right recurrent laryngeal
   c. Left recurrent laryngeal
   d. Left phrenic
4. What is the probable cause of the hoarseness?
   a. Mycotic aortic aneurysm
   b. Tumor recurrence with mediastinal adenopathy
   c. Non-Hodgkin's lymphoma
   d. Fibrosing mediastinitis

Case 56

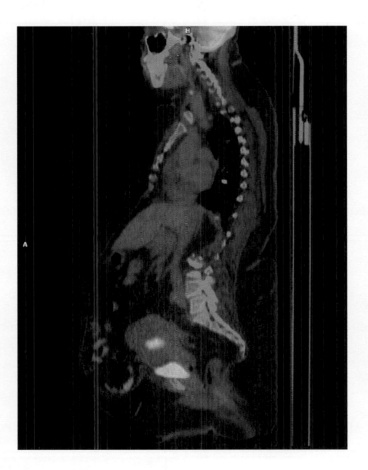

1. Which of the following statements regarding FDG PET/CT in the management of endometrial cancer is correct?
   a. FDG PET/CT is superior to other imaging modalities in the detection and local staging of endometrial cancer.
   b. FDG PET/CT is generally inferior to contrast-enhanced CT and MRI for detecting distant metastasis in advanced stage patients.
   c. FDG PET/CT is the best tool to evaluate for involvement of the cervix.
   d. FDG PET/CT is effective in surveillance of patients for recurrent disease.
2. Risk factors for endometrial cancer include all of the following EXCEPT:
   a. Obesity
   b. Birth control pill
   c. Polycystic ovarian syndrome
   d. Tamoxifen
3. Fused PET/CT images of the endometrium show focal increased uptake in the endometrial cavity with a SUV_{max} of 12. Biopsy shows grade 3 endometrioid adenocarcinoma. Other images (not shown) demonstrate an FDG-avid (SUV_{max} 8) inguinal lymph node, which was subject to biopsy and was positive for tumor. Which of the following corresponds to the correct staging?
   a. Stage I
   b. Stage II
   c. Stage III
   d. Stage IV
4. All of the following are aggressive subtypes of endometrial cancer EXCEPT:
   a. High-grade endometrioid
   b. Clear cell
   c. Serous papillary subtypes
   d. Mucinous

Case 57

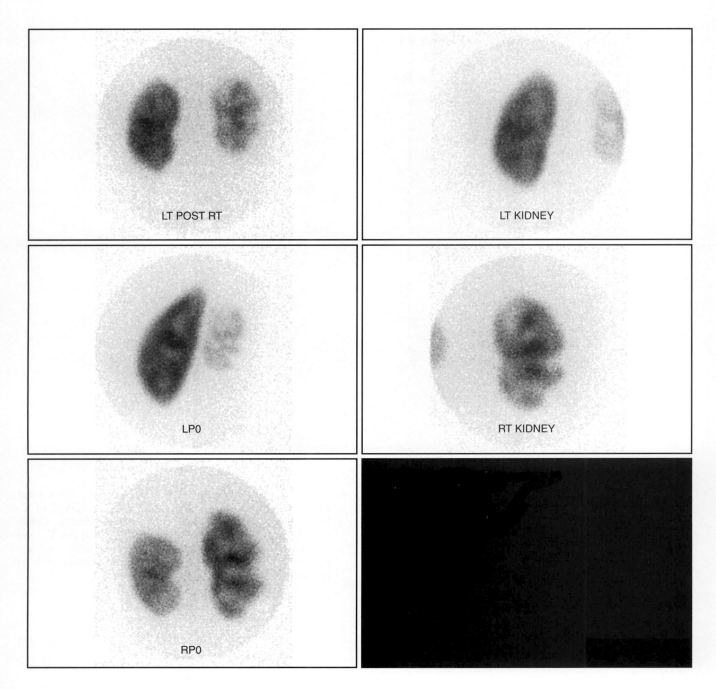

LT POST RT

LT KIDNEY

LPO

RT KIDNEY

RPO

1. Which radiopharmaceutical is utilized in the study?
   a. Tc-99m DTPA
   b. Tc-99m dimercaptosuccinic acid (DMSA)
   c. Tc-99m mercaptoacetyltriglycine (MAG3)
   d. I-131 hippuran
2. Optimal imaging time after injection is (choose the best answer)?
   a. Immediate
   b. 20-30 minutes
   c. 2 hours
   d. 6 hours

3. What kind of collimator has been used to acquire some of the images shown?
   a. Pinhole
   b. Slanthole
   c. Fanbeam
   d. Diverging
4. What is the relevant finding shown in the study?
   a. Abnormal left kidney, hydronephrosis
   b. Abnormal right kidney, scarring
   c. Abnormal left kidney, scarring
   d. Abnormal right kidney, hydronephrosis

Case 58

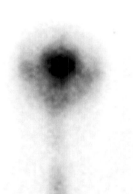

A

B

1. What radiopharmaceutical is utilized in the scan?
   a. Tc-99m DTPA
   b. Tc-99m DMSA
   c. In-111 DTPA
   d. Tc-99m hexamethylpropyleneamine oxime (HMPAO)
2. Where is the radiopharmaceutical injected?
   a. Lateral ventricle
   b. Cisterna magna
   c. Thoracic subarachnoid space
   d. Lumbar subarachnoid space

3. The planar images were obtained 24 hours after injection of the radiopharmaceutical. This appearance is consistent with which of the following?
   a. Normal
   b. Noncommunicating hydrocephalus
   c. Cerebral atrophy
   d. Communicating hydrocephalus
4. All of the following can be associated with the etiology depicted in the scan EXCEPT:
   a. Ataxia
   b. Anosmia
   c. Urinary incontinence
   d. Dementia

Case 59

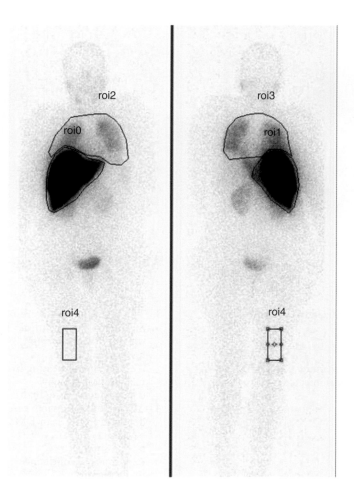

Anterior and posterior planar images from a nuclear medicine study performed in a patient with hepatocellular carcinoma are shown. The study was performed as part of pretherapy planning before treatment with yttrium-90 (Y-90) microspheres.

1. What is the radiopharmaceutical utilized in the study?
   a. Tc-99m Xenon
   b. Tc-99m MAA
   c. Tc-99m SC
   d. In-111 WBC
2. How is the tracer delivered?
   a. Via an antecubital vein
   b. Via the common femoral vein
   c. Via the hepatic artery
   d. Via the hepatic vein

3. What shunt percentage is considered an absolute contraindication to microsphere-based Y-90 treatment:
   a. 5%
   b. 10%
   c. 20%
   d. 50%
4. The examination shows radionuclide activity in the regions of interest in the liver and lungs. What other area of interest is important to observe the presence or absence of uptake?
   a. Brain
   b. Spleen
   c. Gastrointestinal system
   d. Heart

Case 60

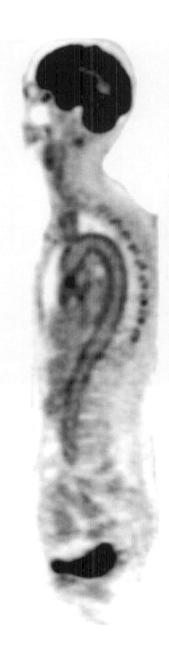

1. The sagittal view of the aorta from an F-18 FDG PET study is shown. What is the most likely diagnosis?
   a. Large vessel vasculitis
   b. Atherosclerosis
   c. Graft infection
   d. Aortic dissection
2. The patient is a 55-year-old male with fever, elevated erythrocyte sedimentation rate (ESR), myalgia, and malaise and no previous history of vascular surgery. He complains of temporal tenderness and jaw claudication. Which of the following is the most likely diagnosis?
   a. Polyarteritis nodosa
   b. Takayasu's arteritis
   c. Giant cell arteritis
   d. Systemic lupus erythematosus
3. What is the clinical utility FDG PET/CT in the management of vasculitis?
   a. Identification of areas to biopsy
   b. Response to therapy
   c. Extent of vessel involvement
   d. All of the above
4. What limits the role of PET/CT in the diagnosis of medium- and small-vessel vasculitis?
   a. Misregistration
   b. Brown fat
   c. Limited resolution
   d. Truncation

Case 61

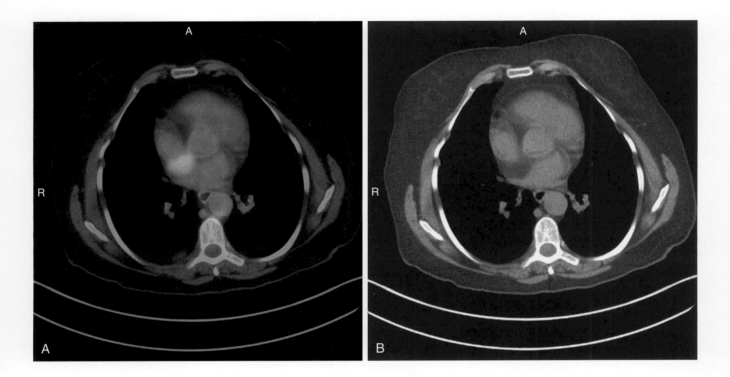

1. CT and fused images of the heart from an F-18-FDG PET/CT scan are shown in a patient being staged for colon cancer. The activity shown on the fused image is localizing to what structure?
   a. Left atrium
   b. Crista terminalis
   c. Right atrial appendage
   d. Interatrial septum
2. Differential considerations for this lesion include all of the following EXCEPT:
   a. Myxoma
   b. Liposarcoma
   c. Lipomatous hypertrophy of the interatrial septum
   d. Arrhythmogenic right ventricular dysplasia (ARVD)

3. All of the following are correct regarding the entity depicted EXCEPT:
   a. Commonly asymptomatic
   b. May present as obstructive right atrial mass
   c. Prevalence increases with age and body mass index
   d. Involves the fossa ovalis
4. Variable FDG uptake in this entity is postulated to be caused by which of the following:
   a. Variable trace amounts of skeletal muscle
   b. Variable amounts of brown fat
   c. Variable amounts of malignant cells
   d. Variable degrees of tissue repair

Case 62

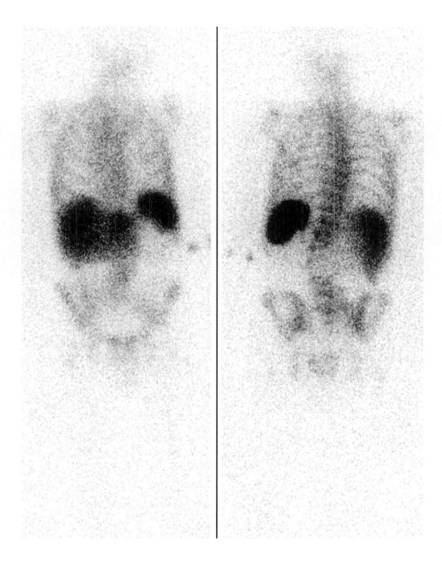

1. All of the following radiopharmaceuticals show physiologic distribution to the liver and spleen with spleen more avid than the liver EXCEPT:
   a. In-111 pentetreotide
   b. In-111 WBC
   c. Gallium-67 (Ga-67) citrate
   d. Tc-99m–labeled RBC
2. With an In-111 WBC study (as shown in the case) to look for infection/inflammation, when is whole body imaging routinely performed?
   a. Immediate and 4 hours
   b. 4 hours and 24 hours
   c. 24 hours and 48 hours
   d. 24 hours
3. The routine-whole body images demonstrate lumbar photopenia on the posterior planar image. All of the following are potential etiologies for the lumbar photopenia EXCEPT:
   a. Vertebral osteomyelitis
   b. Tumor
   c. Paget's disease
   d. Marrow hyperplasia
4. Which group of cells have the highest density of radiolabeling?
   a. Lymphocytes
   b. Basophils
   c. Neutrophils
   d. Platelets

Case 63

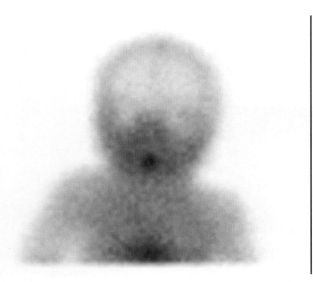

1. A 6-year-old girl complained of dysphagia and was referred for scintigraphy by her physician after physical examination revealed a neck mass. What radiopharmaceutical was utilized in the study?
   a. Tc-99m pertechnetate
   b. Tc-99m DTPA
   c. Tc-99m DMSA
   d. I-131
2. Where is the uptake?
   a. Thyroid bed
   b. Base of tongue
   c. Larynx
   d. Esophagus
3. What is the diagnosis?
   a. Thyroglossal duct cyst
   b. Lymphadenopathy
   c. Ectopic thyroid
   d. Hemangioma
4. Treatment for this entity includes:
   a. Surgery
   b. Radioiodine
   c. Medical therapy
   d. All of the above

Case 64

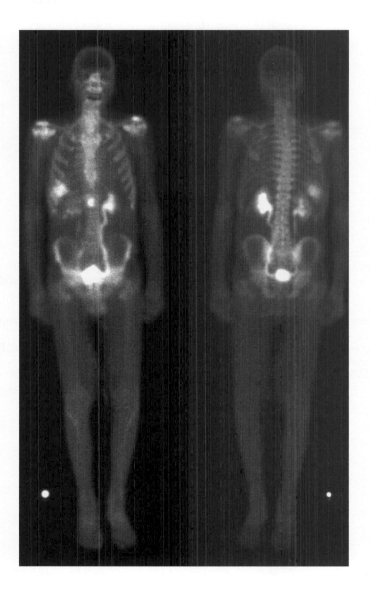

1. The two abnormal foci of tracer uptake on this Tc-99m MDP bone scan could be in all of the following locations EXCEPT:
   a. Liver only
   b. Liver and pancreas
   c. Liver and abdominal lymph node
   d. Liver and vertebral body
2. Which of the following usually presents as focal/heterogeneous hepatic uptake on a Tc-99m MDP bone scan?
   a. Hepatitis
   b. Metastatic carcinoma
   c. Recent administration of other radiopharmaceuticals
   d. Impurities in the radiopharmaceutical preparation

3. Which is a cause of improper preparation of the radiopharmaceutical, Tc-99m – MDP, which may result in hepatic uptake on the bone scan?
   a. Excess molybdenum-99 (Mo-99) in the eluate.
   b. Excess alumina chemical impurity, resulting in colloid formation
   c. Radiochemical impurity with reduction states of + 4, + 5, or + 6
   d. Excessive oxygen in the reaction vial during radiolabeling
4. All of the following physiologic mechanisms may contribute to localization of Tc-99m – MDP in extraosseous metastatic disease on bone scan EXCEPT:
   a. Increased regional blood flow
   b. Increased tissue calcium
   c. Increased tissue magnesium
   d. Increased vascular permeability

Case 65

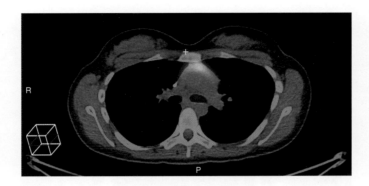

1. An axial image from an F-18 FDG PET/CT scan in a 22-year-old patient after chemotherapy for treatment of lymphoma is shown. Differential considerations include all of the following EXCEPT:
   a. Thymic rebound
   b. Recurrent lymphoma
   c. Vascular blood pool activity
   d. Thymoma
2. The uptake shown is the only region of hypermetabolic activity in the patient who finished chemotherapy 8 months ago. The SUV_{max} of the lesion is 2.8. What is the most likely diagnosis?
   a. Thymic rebound
   b. Recurrent lymphoma

   c. Normal thymus
   d. Thymic carcinoma
3. Which of the following features of the lesion may help distinguish normal thymus/thymic rebound from malignant etiologies?
   a. Diffuse enlargement
   b. Presence of fat
   c. Homogenous enhancement
   d. All of the above
4. In what age group is normal, FDG-avid thymic activity seen?
   a. Less than 20 years
   b. 20–30 years
   c. 30–40 years
   d. 50 years and older

Case 66

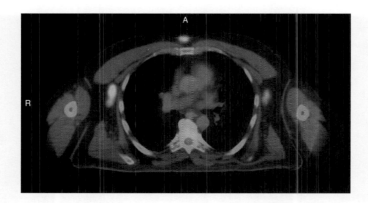

A patient presents for initial staging with F-18 FDG PET/CT for melanoma.

1. All of the following are prognostic factors for localized cutaneous melanoma EXCEPT:
   a. Tumor thickness
   b. Sentinel lymph node status
   c. Ulceration
   d. SUV_{max}

2. Sentinel lymph node biopsy (SLNB) is considered the standard of care in which of the following patients diagnosed with malignant melanoma?
   a. Patients with stage I or II disease, particularly those with an intermediate Breslow thickness, between 1 and 4 mm
   b. Patients with confirmed American Joint Committee on Cancer (AJCC) stage III disease
   c. Patients with head and neck tumor, regardless of stage
   d. Patients with metastatic disease with an unknown primary

3. Which of the following statements regarding role of FDG PET/CT in staging melanoma is true?
   a. FDG PET/CT staging may alter management in approximately 70% of patients with known or suspected metastases.
   b. FDG PET/CT is cost effective in patients with AJCC stage I or II disease.
   c. FDG PET/CT is superior to MRI and CT in the staging of stage III and IV disease.
   d. FDG PET/CT is complementary to MRI and CT in detection of recurrent disease.

4. In the patient depicted in the case, based on the fused PET/CT image, what is the stage of the tumor?
   a. Stage I
   b. Stage II
   c. Stage III
   d. Stage IV

Case 67

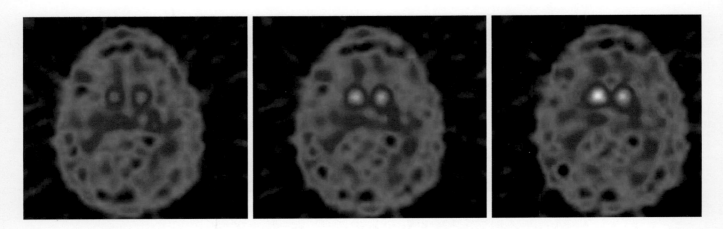

1. What is the radiopharmaceutical utilized in the scan?
   a. Tc-99m HMPAO
   b. F-18 FDG
   c. I-123 ioflupane
   d. Thallium-201 (Tl-201)
2. The molecular imaging agent shown demonstrates the location and concentration of which the following in the brain?
   a. Dopamine transporter
   b. Vesicular monoamine transporter
   c. Aromatic amino acid decarboxylase
   d. L-dopa
3. Which imaging technique is utilized?
   a. PET
   b. Single photon emission computed tomography (SPECT)
   c. MRI
   d. Optical imaging
4. For the patient depicted in the scan, all of the following disorders are possible EXCEPT:
   a. Essential tremor
   b. Progressive supranuclear palsy
   c. Idiopathic Parkinson's disease
   d. Multiple system atrophy

Case 68

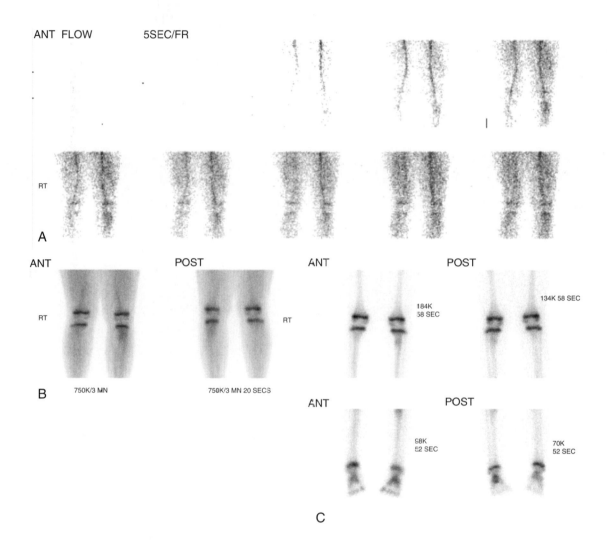

ANT FLOW   5SEC/FR

RT

A

ANT   POST   ANT   POST

RT   RT   184K 58 SEC   134K 58 SEC

B   750K/3 MN   750K/3 MN 20 SECS

ANT   POST

98K 52 SEC   70K 52 SEC

C

A 6-year-old girl presents with left lower extremity pain, no fever, and normal WBC count. She was recently treated with oral antibiotics for presumed osteomyelitis a few weeks earlier.

1. Which organ receives the highest radiation dose in a three-phase bone scan?
   a. Skeleton
   b. Marrow
   c. Kidneys
   d. Bladder

2. All of the following may be hot on all three phases of a bone scan EXCEPT:
   a. Acute fracture
   b. Cellulitis
   c. Osteomyelitis
   d. Neuropathic joint

3. The infectious disease team, after reviewing the laboratory data, the clinical history, and the radiographs, does not think the patient has osteomyelitis. The patient does complain of increased pain at night, which is alleviated by ibuprofen. Which of the following entities do you suspect?
   a. Osteoblastoma
   b. Osteosarcoma
   c. Stress fracture
   d. Osteoid osteoma

4. What is the next test you would recommend?
   a. In-111 WBC
   b. Tc-99 SC
   c. CT
   d. F-18 FDG PET/CT

Case 69

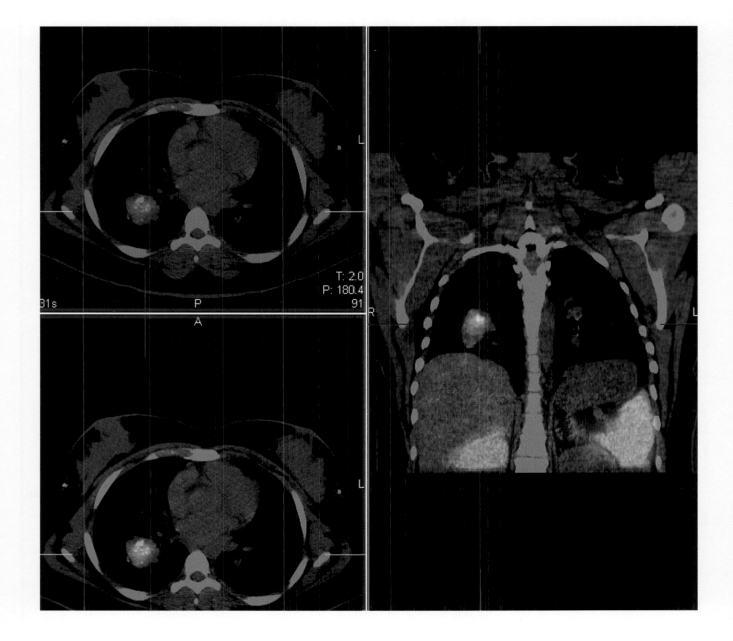

1. The CT image shows a lobulated right perihilar lung mass with coarse calcification. The differential diagnosis based on the CT images alone includes all of the following EXCEPT:
   a. Primary pulmonary carcinoma
   b. Bronchopulmonary carcinoid
   c. Hamartoma
   d. Granuloma

2. The patient states she previously had a PET/CT examination to evaluate the finding. You find the report in the patient's folder, and the nodule was noted to have low-grade activity on the PET/CT scan, SUV_{max} 1.5, and was noted to be indeterminate for malignancy. Bronchoscopy noted an endoluminal component to the lesion. What is your favored diagnosis?
   a. Primary pulmonary carcinoma
   b. Bronchopulmonary carcinoid
   c. Hamartoma
   d. Mucoepidermoid carcinoma

3. What is the study being performed?
   a. F-18 FDG PET/CT
   b. F-18 sodium fluoride (NaF) PET/CT
   c. In-111 Octreoscan (pentetreotide) SPECT/CT
   d. I-123 MIBG

4. In the study being performed, what is the preferred imaging time?
   a. 1 hour
   b. 12 hours
   c. 24 hours
   d. 72 hours

Case 70

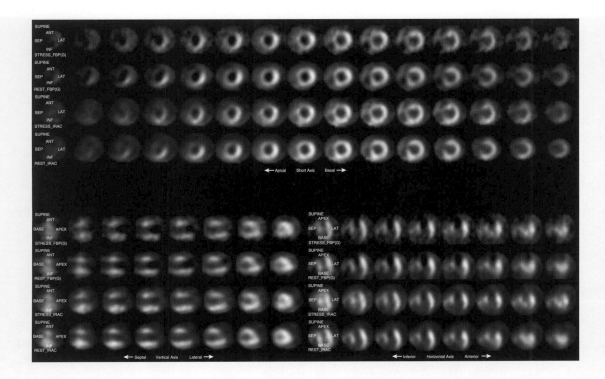

These are images from a rest–stress myocardial perfusion study, including filtered back projection (FBP) images and attenuation corrected (AC) images.

1. What is the finding on this exercise myocardial perfusion study?
   a. Anteroapical septal infarct
   b. Anteroapical septal ischemia
   c. Inferior wall infarct
   d. Inferior wall ischemia
2. To assess for viability, what study would you perform?
   a. Tc-99m sestamibi rest
   b. Tc-99m RBC MUGA
   c. Tc-99m sestamibi stress
   d. F-18 FDG
3. Although not present in this case, what is the clinical significance of transient ischemic dilatation (TID)?
   a. Incomplete exercise
   b. Technical
   c. Three-vessel coronary artery disease
   d. Myocarditis
4. Although not present in this case, in the setting of left bundle branch block, what imaging findings may be seen?
   a. Exercise-induced apical fixed defect
   b. Exercise-induced septal wall reversible defect
   c. Regadenoson-induced apical fixed defect
   d. Regadenoson-induced septal reversible defect

Case 71

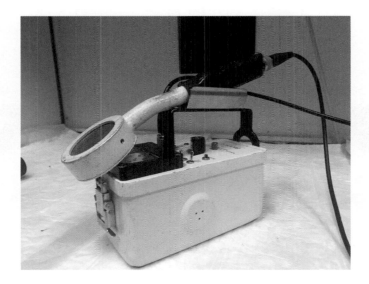

1. What is the name of this instrument?
   a. Geiger-Muller counter
   b. Thyroid probe
   c. Dose calibrator
   d. Well counter
2. What dose of radiation would this instrument be best suited for?
   a. Less than 100 mR/hour
   b. 100–220 mR/hour
   c. 200–500 mR/hour
   d. Greater than 500 mR/hour
3. What best describes the mode of operation for this instrument?
   a. Scintillation detection
   b. Ionization detection
   c. Iterative reconstruction
   d. Photodisintegration
4. What does the gain switch do?
   a. Changes the optimal photopeak to mirror the radionuclide being measured
   b. Turns the instrument on and off
   c. Serves as a multiplier for the number of counts being detected
   d. Increases the volume

Case 72

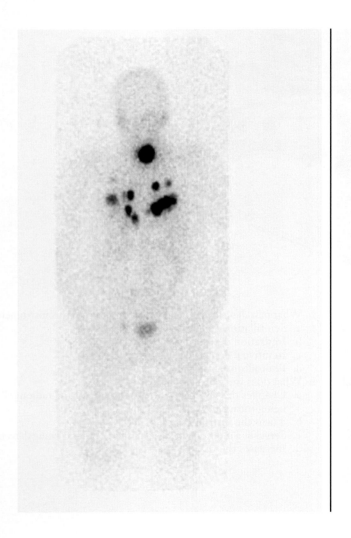 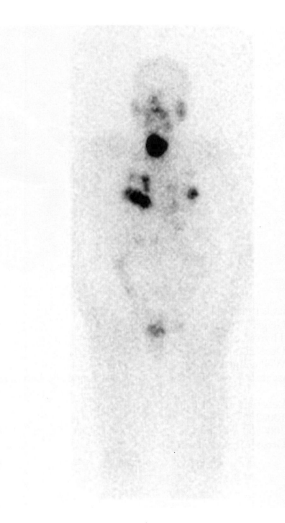

1. What is the likely clinical history?
   a. 40 packs per year smoker
   b. Fever of unknown origin
   c. Palpable thyroid nodule
   d. Dark, irregular mole on the upper back
2. What is the diagnosis?
   a. Lung metastases from thyroid cancer
   b. Multifocal pneumonia
   c. Lung metastases from a colon primary
   d. Bronchiolitis obliterans
3. What dose of I-123 is used for whole body scanning?
   a. 200 μCi
   b. 2 mCi
   c. 15 mCi
   d. 30 mCi
4. What is the therapeutic mechanism for I-131 therapy?
   a. Alpha particle emission
   b. High-energy gamma photons
   c. Beta particle emission
   d. Positron emission

Case 73

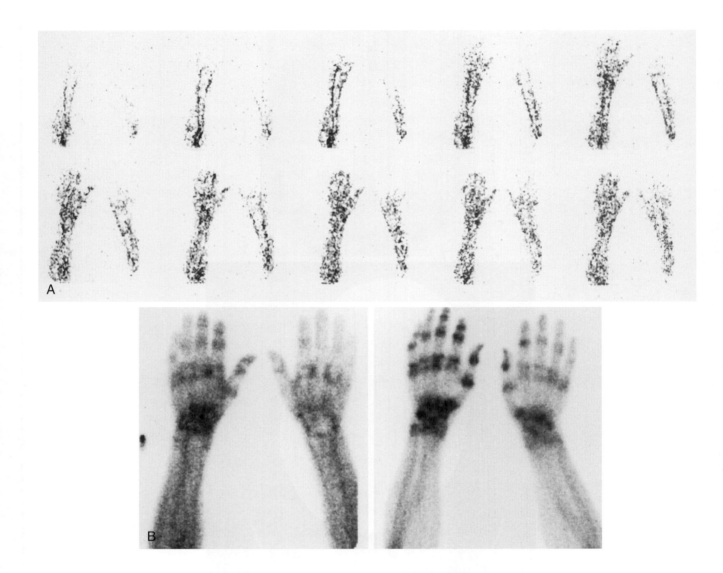

A

B

Images from a three-phase bone scan of the forearms and hands in a patient who presents with extremity pain are shown.

1. Which of the following best describes the findings?
   a. Increased flow and increased blood pool uptake in the left forearm and hand; increased periarticular uptake in the left wrist and hand on delayed images.
   b. Increased flow and increased blood pool uptake in the right forearm and hand; decreased uptake in the left hand on delayed images.
   c. Decreased flow and increased blood pool in the left forearm and hand; increased periarticular uptake in the right wrist and hand
   d. Decreased flow and decreased blood pool uptake in the left forearm and hand; increased periarticular uptake in the right wrist and hand on delayed images.

2. What is the diagnosis?
   a. Cellulitis
   b. Osteomyelitis
   c. Multiple fractures
   d. Complex regional pain syndrome

3. Correlative radiographic findings may show which of the following?
   a. Normal or demineralization
   b. Fractures
   c. Cortical erosions
   d. Periosteal thickening

4. All of the following may be associated with the entity depicted EXCEPT:
   a. Trauma/injury/surgery
   b. Stroke
   c. Myocardial infarction
   d. Pulmonary Infarct

Case 74

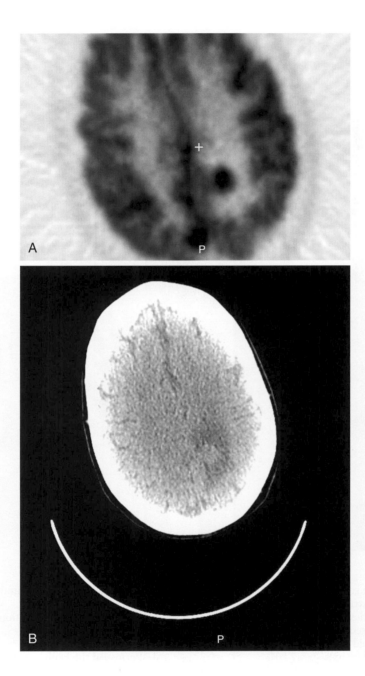

1. What is the most likely diagnosis in a 45-year-old patient with a primary central nervous system (CNS) malignancy?
   a. Low-grade oligodendroglioma
   b. Lymphoma
   c. Ganglioglioma
   d. Metastases
2. What is the most likely histology?
   a. Non-Hodgkin's lymphoma (NHL)
   b. Hodgkin's lymphoma (HD)
   c. Mucosa-associated lymphoid tissue (MALT) lymphoma
   d. Gastrointestinal stromal tumor (GIST)

3. What is the likelihood of systemic disease?
   a. Less than 1%
   b. Less than 10%
   c. 10%–25 %
   d. 50%
4. What is the most likely CNS location of this entity?
   a. Supratentorial, intracranial
   b. Posterior fossa
   c. Spinal cord
   d. Dural

Case 75

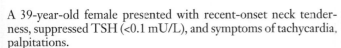

ANTERIOR
14:49:33.0

A 39-year-old female presented with recent-onset neck tenderness, suppressed TSH (<0.1 mU/L), and symptoms of tachycardia, palpitations.

1. All of the following are in the differential for thyrotoxicosis EXCEPT:
   a. Graves' disease
   b. Subacute thyroiditis
   c. Struma ovarii
   d. Follicular adenoma

2. An I-123 radioactive iodine uptake (RAIU) and scan are performed. Which of the following best explains how this test aids in narrowing the differential for this patient with a suppressed serum TSH ?
   a. Elevated RAIU indicates autonomous hyperfunctioning thyroid tissue
   b. Elevated RAIU indicates exogenous sources of ingested thyroid hormone
   c. Decreased RAIU differentiates autoimmune causes from bacterial causes
   d. Decreased RAIU indicates tumors of the pituitary gland causing thyrotoxicosis

3. Given the images shown and a very low RAIU, which of the following is the most likely diagnosis?
   a. Graves' disease
   b. Subacute thyroiditis
   c. Struma ovarii
   d. Metastatic thyroid cancer

4. If the clinical history instead showed that the patient was a 50-year-old health care worker with thyrotoxicosis and undetectable serum thyroglobulin, what would be the likely diagnosis?
   a. Amiodarone toxicity
   b. Pituitary gland tumor
   c. Thyroiditis factitia
   d. Struma ovarii

Case 76

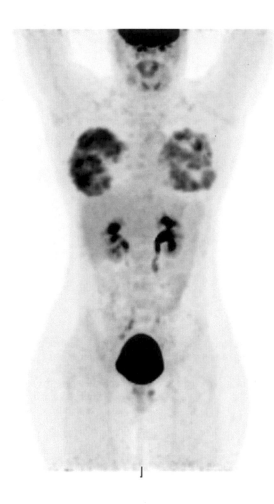

Whole-body maximum-intensity projection (MIP) from an F-18 FDG PET in a female patient for surveillance scan for follow-up of lymphoma is shown.

1. Which of the following descriptions of the findings is most appropriate?
   a. Intense, diffuse symmetric uptake in both breasts.
   b. Low-grade uptake in the anterior bilateral chest well
   c. Intense, heterogeneous uptake in both breasts, mildly asymmetric
   d. Mild heterogeneous uptake in the bilateral intramammary nodes

2. If corresponding CT image shows bilateral innumerable dense lobulated masses in both breasts bilaterally. The patient has a history of cosmetic breast procedure. What is the most likely diagnosis?
   a. Active lactation
   b. Postoperative changes and fat necrosis
   c. Silicone injection granulomas
   d. Bilateral fibroadenomas

3. Corresponding CT image shows dense breast tissue. Patient is postpartum. What is the most likely diagnosis?
   a. Active lactation
   b. Postoperative changes and fat necrosis
   c. Silicone injection granulomas
   d. Bilateral fibroadenomas

4. Which of the following statements regarding FDG and lactation is correct?
   a. Complete cessation of breastfeeding is advised after administration of 18-FDG because greater than 10% of the administered dose may be excreted in breast milk.
   b. Breastfeeding should be stopped for 24 hours after administration of 18-FDG. Breast milk may be expressed after the examination and discarded.
   c. Breastfeeding should not be interrupted, but close contact between mother and child should be limited for 12 hours following injection to reduce the radiation dose that the infant receives from external exposure to radiation emitted by the mother. Breast milk can be expressed and bottle fed to the infant.
   d. Breastfeeding should be stopped for 4 hours after injection of 18-FDG, and breast milk should be pumped and stored during this time to be used later after activity dissipates.

Case 77

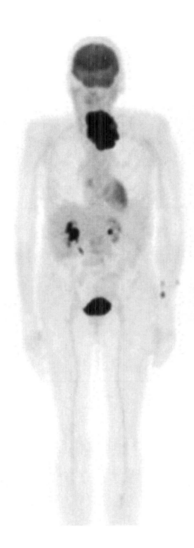

A 78-year-old female presented with rapidly enlarging neck mass and hoarseness.

1. All of the following are in the differential diagnosis of this FDG PET scan EXCEPT:
   a. Anaplastic thyroic carcinoma
   b. Graves' disease
   c. NHL of thyroid
   d. Thyroid-differentiated carcinoma

2. The CT component of the F-18 FDG PET/CT scan (not shown) reveals homogeneous density of the mass, no calcification, adjacent lymphadenopathy, and no gross invasion of adjacent structures. The patient is noted to have a history of chronic lymphocytic thyroiditis. What is the most likely diagnosis?
   a. Anaplastic thyroic carcinoma
   b. Graves' disease
   c. NHL of the thyroid
   d. Thyroid differentiated carcinoma

3. How is this entity staged?
   a. AJCC, TNM: always T4
   b. Ann Arbor System
   c. Lugano's Classification
   d. Deauville's five-point scale

4. Which treatment is not indicated in the setting of a patent airway?
   a. Rituximab
   b. Radiation
   c. Chemotherapy
   d. Thyroidectomy

Case 78

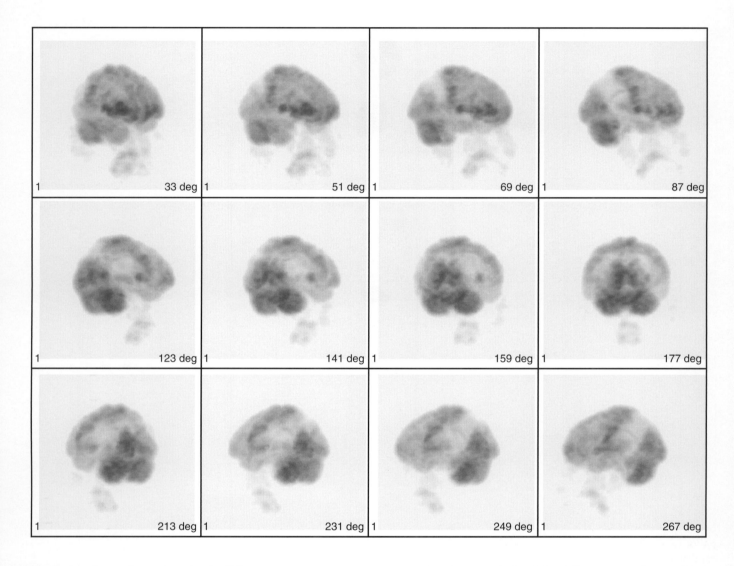

MIP images from a brain F-18 FDG PET scan in a patient presenting with memory difficulties are shown.

1. Which of the following best describes the findings?
   a. Hypermetabolism in the bilateral frontal lobes and occipital lobes
   b. Hypometabolism in the bilateral parietal and temporal lobes, including the posterior cingulate gyrus with relative sparing of the frontal and occipital lobes
   c. Hypometabolism in the bilateral temporal and frontal lobes, with relative sparing of the basal ganglia
   d. Focal hypermetabolism in the right frontal lobe
2. In diffuse Lewy body disease, which of the following is a distinguishing feature on FDG PET?
   a. Hypometabolism in the cingulate gyrus
   b. Hypometabolism in the thalamus
   c. Hypometabolism in the occipital lobe
   d. Hypermetabolism in the hippocampus
3. In Pick's disease, which of the following is a distinguishing feature on FDG-PET?
   a. Hypometabolism in the posterior cingulate gyrus
   b. Hypometabolism in the thalamus
   c. Hypometabolism in the frontal and temporal lobe, with involvement of the anterior cingulate cortex
   d. Hypermetabolism in the hippocampus
4. What is the most likely diagnosis based on the scan shown?
   a. Alzheimer's dementia
   b. Diffuse Lewy body disease
   c. Frontotemporal dementia
   d. Vascular dementia

Case 79

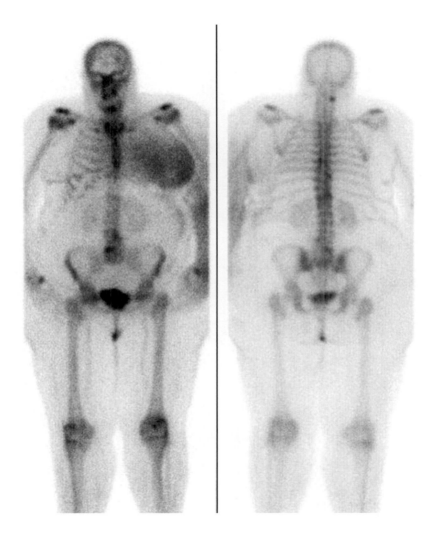

1. This bone scan shows abnormal soft uptake in the left chest which localizes to which of the following structures?
   a. Shoulder
   b. Breast
   c. Axilla
   d. Lung
2. All of the following are included in the differential of the soft tissue uptake EXCEPT:
   a. Dystrophic calcification
   b. Rhabdomyolysis
   c. Neoplasm
   d. Fibrocystic disease
3. Other abnormal areas of skeletal uptake on the bone scan include all of the following EXCEPT the:
   a. Sternum
   b. Thoracic spine
   c. Knees
   d. Lumbar spine
4. What study would you recommend for further evaluation of the skeletal findings and further staging?
   a. MRI of cervical, thoracic, and lumbar spine, without contrast
   b. CT of neck, chest, abdomen, and pelvis
   c. Radiography of spine and chest
   d. FDG PET/CT, from skull base to thigh

Case 80

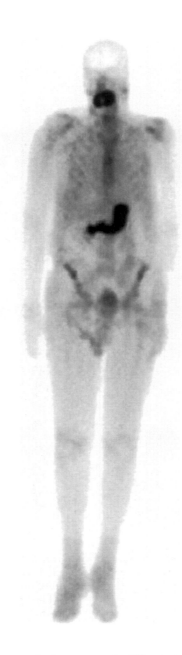

A whole-body anterior planar image from a bone scan is shown.

1. Where is the abnormal uptake on this whole body Tc-99m MDP bone scan?
   a. Bones
   b. Kidneys
   c. Stomach and oral cavity
   d. Lung
2. What is the likely cause of this uptake?
   a. Free Tc-99m pertechnetate in the prepared radiopharmaceutical
   b. Recent prior Tc-99m liver spleen scan
   c. Hypercalcemia
   d. Diffuse gastric cancer

3. What is the next step of investigation?
   a. Send patient's blood for chemistry panel and complete blood cell count (CBC)
   b. Recommend contrast-enhanced abdominal CT scan
   c. Recommend upper endoscopy
   d. None of the above
4. What is the reducing agent used with Tc-99m to form Tc-99m MDP?
   a. Lithium
   b. Stannous ion
   c. Copper
   d. Silver

Case 81

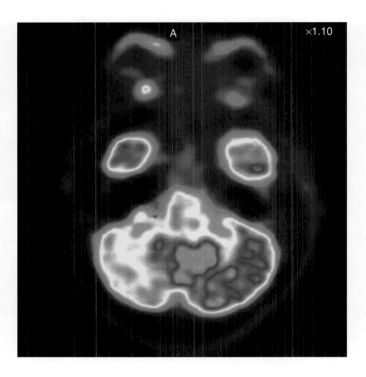

1. What is the diagnosis based on this brain scan in a patient with a left-sided frontal lobe mass (not pictured)?
   a. Posterior fossa brain tumor
   b. Crossed cerebellar diaschisis
   c. Extra-axial lesion
   d. Normal scan
2. What is the radiopharmaceutical?
   a. Tc-99m DTPA
   b. F-18 FDG
   c. F-18 NaF
   d. Tc-99m MDP

3. What is the radiopharmaceutical uptake time?
   a. 10 minutes
   b. 30 minutes
   c. 60 minutes
   d. 180 minutes
4. What are the possible etiologies for this finding?
   a. Infarct
   b. Primary brain tumor
   c. Postoperative changes
   d. All of the above

Case 82

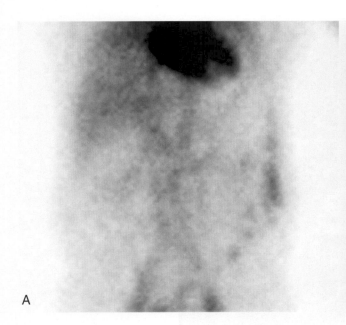

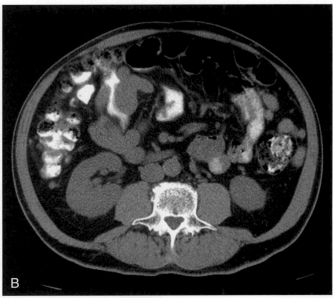

1. What is the radiopharmaceutical?
   a. Tc-99m MDP
   b. Tc-99m RBC
   c. Tc-99m DTPA
   d. Tc-99m DSMA
2. What is the diagnosis?
   a. Active bleed
   b. Splenosis
   c. Ectatic vasculature
   d. Angiodysplasia

3. What is the most common cause of this finding?
   a. Metastatic disease
   b. Congenital
   c. Infection
   d. Trauma
4. How would you differentiate this finding from a GI bleed?
   a. GI bleed will demonstrate ante(retro)grade movement of radiotracer uptake.
   b. Splenosis will demonstrate ante(retro)grade movement of radiotracer uptake.
   c. GI bleed will demonstrate low level of uptake.
   d. Splenosis will demonstrate high level of uptake.

Case 83

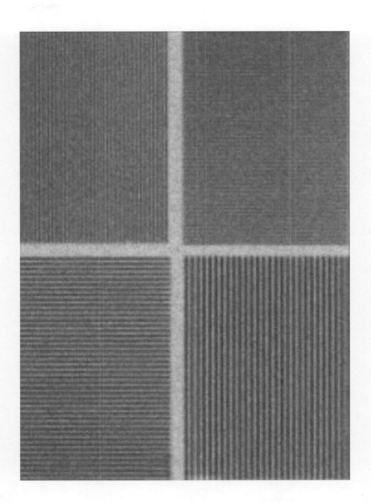

1. What is this image?
   a. Intrinsic flood image
   b. Four-quadrant bar image
   c. Extrinsic flood image
   d. Uniformity image
2. How often is this image acquired?
   a. Daily
   b. Weekly
   c. Monthly
   d. Annually

3. What does this image assess?
   a. Uniformity and linearity
   b. Uniformity and spatial resolution
   c. Energy resolution and linearity
   d. Linearity and spatial resolution
4. What are the bars composed of ?
   a. Tc-99m
   b. Lead
   c. Cobalt-157 (Co-157)
   d. I-123

Case 84

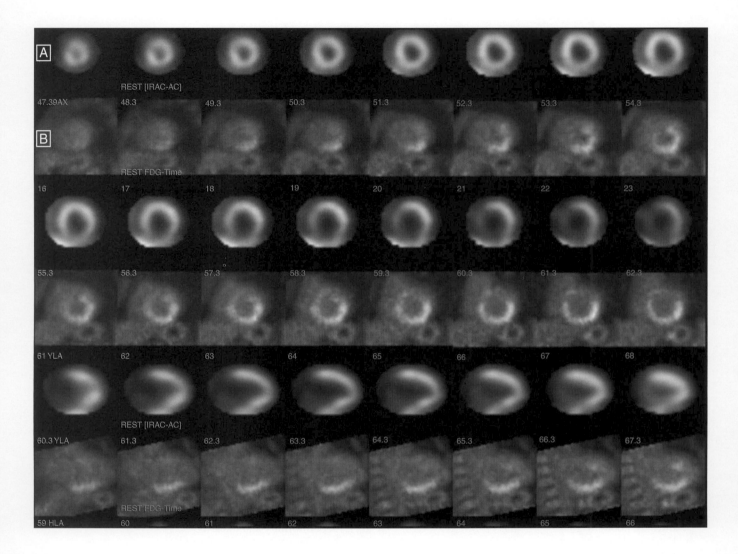

These are cardiac PET/CT scans, including a perfusion scan (top row) and an FDG scan (bottom row).

1. Where is the perfusion abnormality?
   a. Anterior wall
   b. Anterolateral wall
   c. Inferior/inferoseptal wall
   d. Lateral wall
2. Why is this test performed?
   a. To evaluate for myocardial infarct
   b. To evaluate for myocardial ischemia
   c. To evaluate for hibernating myocardium
   d. To quantify ejection fraction (EF)
3. What are the clinical implications of FDG uptake?
   a. Revascularization is not indicated
   b. Revascularization may be indicated
   c. Steroid should be added to reduce inflammation
   d. No need for steroid therapy
4. What is the rationale for using FDG?
   a. Hibernating myocardium will preferentially use fatty acids for metabolism
   b. Hibernating myocardium will preferentially use glucose for metabolism
   c. Hibernating myocardium will take up FDG because of significant inflammation
   d. Hibernating myocardium will not take up FDG because of significant inflammation

Case 85

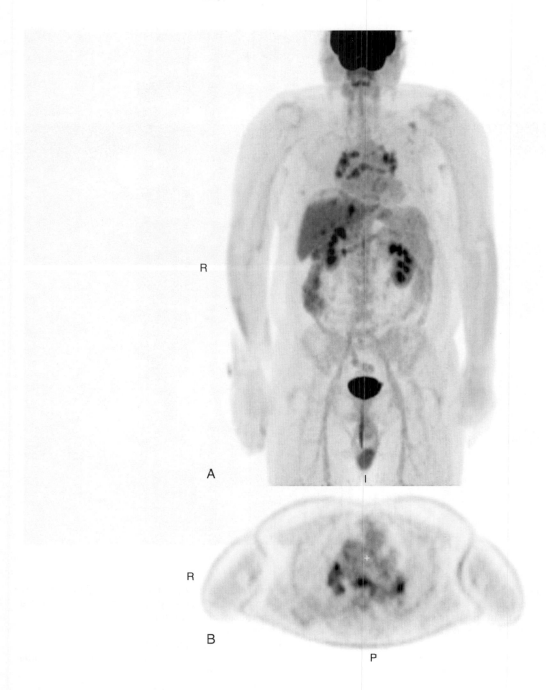

1. What is the radiopharmaceutical?
   a. F-18 FDG
   b. Tc-99m MDP
   c. I-123 MIBG
   d. F-18 NaF
2. What is the most likely etiology for these findings in a patient with evidence of interstitial lung disease on chest radiography?
   a. Lymphoma
   b. Granulomatous disease
   c. Chronic lymphocytic lymphoma (CLL)
   d. Normal physiologic uptake
3. What is the histologic hallmark of sarcoidosis?
   a. Noncaseating granulomas
   b. Caseating granulomas
   c. Plaque formation
   d. Neurofibrillary tangles
4. What is the first-line therapy for sarcoidosis?
   a. Chemotherapy
   b. Radiation
   c. Immunotherapy
   d. Steroids

Case 86

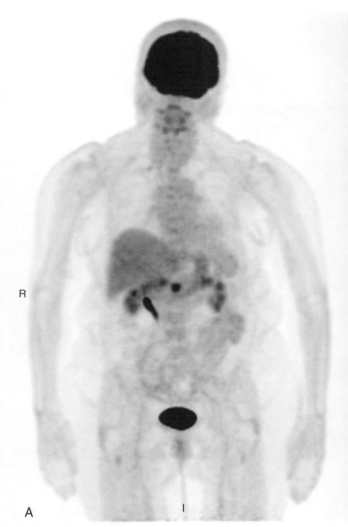

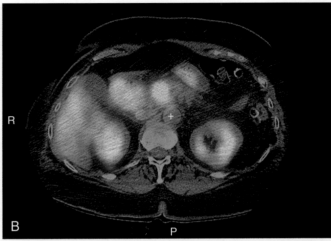

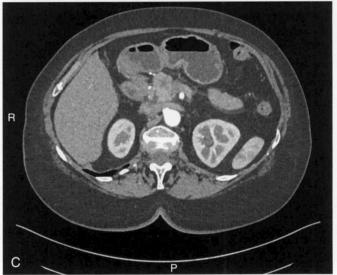

Multiple images from a F-18 FDG PET/CT scan with axial and fused images at the level of the pancreas are shown.

1. The SUV_{max} of the mass in the head of the pancreas is approximately 8. All of the following are considered in the differential EXCEPT:
   a. Islet cell tumor
   b. Poorly differentiated neuroendocrine tumor
   c. Adenocarcinoma
   d. Lymphoma

2. Which of the following best describes the role of FDG PET/CT in the management of pancreatic adenocarcinoma?
   a. FDG PET/CT is superior to CT and MRI for initial staging of disease.
   b. FDG PET/CT is modality of choice in determination of tumor resectability.
   c. FDG PET/CT is recommended for annual surveillance in posttreatment patients.
   d. FDG PET/CT is accurate at predicting survival based on the SUV_{max} of the tumor.

3. Which of the following is a limitation of PET/CT that may lead to false-positive or false-negative findings in the evaluation of pancreatic adenocarcinoma?
   a. Spatial resolution
   b. Partial volume averaging in small lesions
   c. Inflammatory uptake related to treatment (surgery, radiation, stent placement)
   d. All of the above

4. Common sites of distant metastatic spread of pancreatic adenocarcinoma include all of the following EXCEPT the:
   a. Liver
   b. Peritoneum
   c. Perineural celiac and mesenteric plexuses
   d. Pericardium

Case 87

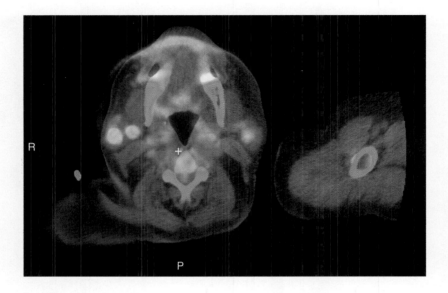

A single fused image from a PET/CT scan at the level of the mandible in a patient being evaluated for a single pulmonary nodule is shown.

1. Where is the abnormal uptake?
   a. Subcutaneous fat of the neck
   b. Jugulodigastric lymph nodes
   c. Sternocleidomastoid muscle
   d. Parotid gland
2. Which of the following choices best describes the findings?
   a. Bilateral symmetric uptake in the masseter muscles
   b. Bilateral uptake in the jugulodigastric lymph nodes
   c. Unilateral hypermetabolism in the right sternocleidomastoid muscle
   d. Bilateral multifocal hypermetabolic activity in the parotid glands

3. All of the following are differential considerations EXCEPT:
   a. Hypermetabolic benign brown fat
   b. Warthin's tumor
   c. Parotid benign mixed tumor
   d. Lymphoma
4. The patient's medical history states that he is a 30-pack-year smoker. What is the most likely diagnosis?
   a. Focal Infection
   b. Warthin's tumor
   c. Parotid benign mixed tumor
   d. Lymphoma

Case 88

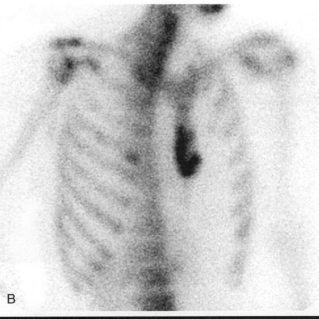

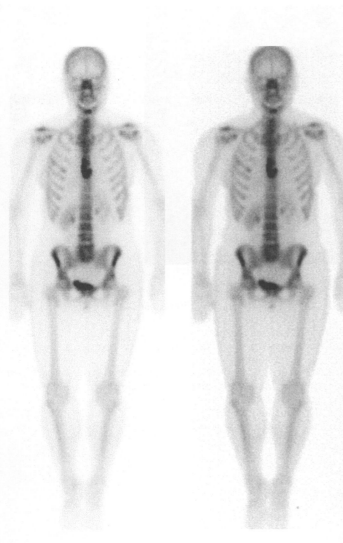

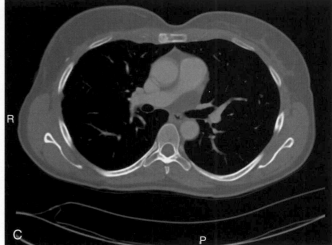

A

B

C

R   P

1. What is the likely diagnosis?
   a. Prostate cancer
   b. Breast cancer
   c. Lung cancer
   d. Pancreatic cancer
2. What is the radiopharmaceutical?
   a. Tc-99m mebrofenin
   b. Tc-99m DTPA
   c. Tc-99m MDP
   d. F-18 FDG

3. The most common etiology for sternal uptake is:
   a. Physiologic sternomanubrial uptake
   b. Previous trauma
   c. Metastasis
   d. Osteoblastoma
4. What is the likelihood that this finding represents metastases in a patient with history of breast cancer?
   a. Less than 10%
   b. 10%–20%
   c. 20%–50%
   d. Approximately 80%

Case 89

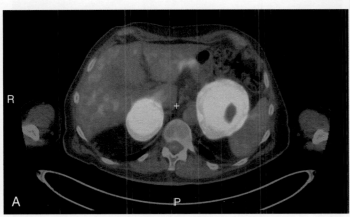

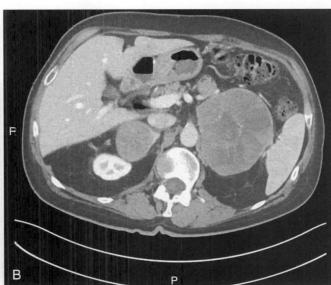

A fused F-18 FDG PET/CT image and an axial contrast-enhanced CT scan at the level of the adrenal glands are shown.

1. The patient has a history of melanoma. What is the most likely diagnosis?
   a. Bilateral adrenal cortical carcinomas
   b. Bilateral adrenal metastases
   c. Bilateral adrenal adenomas
   d. Bilateral adrenal tuberculosis

2. The patient has a history of multiple endocrine neoplasia type 2A (MEN 2A). What is the most likely diagnosis?
   a. Bilateral adrenal cortical carcinoma
   b. Bilateral adrenal metastases
   c. Bilateral adrenal lymphoma
   d. Bilateral adrenal pheochromocytoma

3. The patient has recently immigrated to North America and presents with a history of fatigue, weakness, nausea, vomiting, and increasing skin pigmentation over recent months. No history of malignancy. What is the most likely diagnosis?
   a. Bilateral adrenal cortical carcinoma
   b. Bilateral adrenal tuberculosis
   c. Bilateral adrenal adenomas
   d. Bilateral adrenal pheochromocytoma

4. All of the following primary tumors tend to metastasize to the adrenal glands, EXCEPT:
   a. Lung cancer
   b. Melanoma
   c. Prostate cancer
   d. Renal cell carcinoma

Case 90

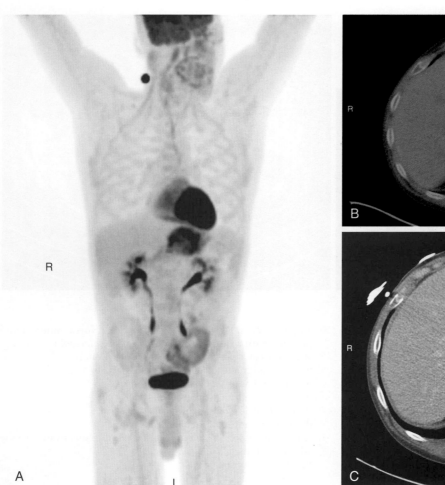

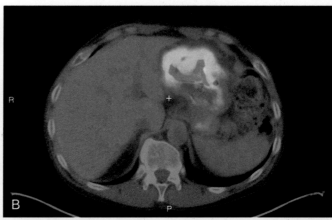

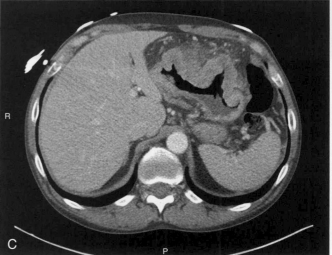

Multiple images from an F-18 FDG PET/CT scan performed for initial evaluation of gastric cancer are shown.

1. Where is the abnormal uptake?
   a. Gastroesophageal junction
   b. Posterior gastric fundus, with left adrenal metastasis
   c. Anterior gastric body, with penetration of the serosa
   d. Gastric cardia, with peritoneal uptake in left lower pelvis

2. What is the probable histologic subtype of the tumor?
   a. Mucinous carcinoma
   b. Signet cell ring carcinoma
   c. MALT lymphoma
   d. Intestinal type adenocarcinoma

3. All of the following are risk factors for the development of gastric cancer EXCEPT:
   a. Eosinophilic gastritis
   b. *Helicobacter pylori* infection
   c. Pernicious anemia
   d. Diet heavy in nitrates and nitrites

4. What is a common site for metastatic disease?
   a. Liver
   b. Lung
   c. Peritoneum
   d. All of the above

Case 91

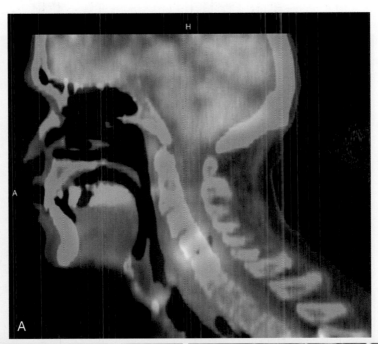

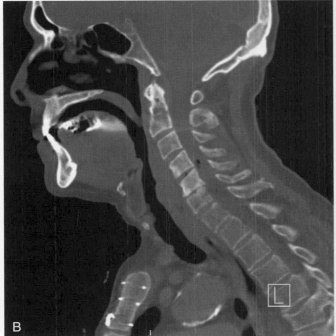

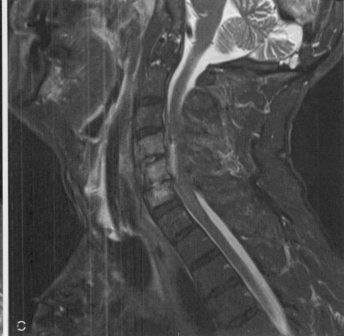

Images from a patient with new-onset neck pain are shown.

1. What is the salient finding in the FDG PET/CT?
   a. Degenerative changes in the cervical spine
   b. FDG avidity in the cervical spine suspicious for infection or metastases
   c. Esophageal inflammatory changes
   d. Normal physiologic activity likely related to recent ingestion of food

2. The patient subsequently underwent MRI. What is your diagnosis?
   a. Metastases to cervical spine
   b. Discitis/osteomyelitis with epidural abscess
   c. Degenerative changes
   d. Spinal cord malignancy

3. What is the appropriate treatment if patient has neurologic deficits, as revealed by the examination?
   a. Low-dose steroids
   b. Oral antibiotics
   c. Surgery
   d. Chemotherapy

4. What is the imaging protocol for F-18 FDG evaluation of infections?
   a. Same as oncologic F-18 FDG PET/CT
   b. No need to be NPO (nothing by mouth)
   c. Give intravenous (IV) insulin before imaging to enhance uptake
   d. Image at 4 hours after injection

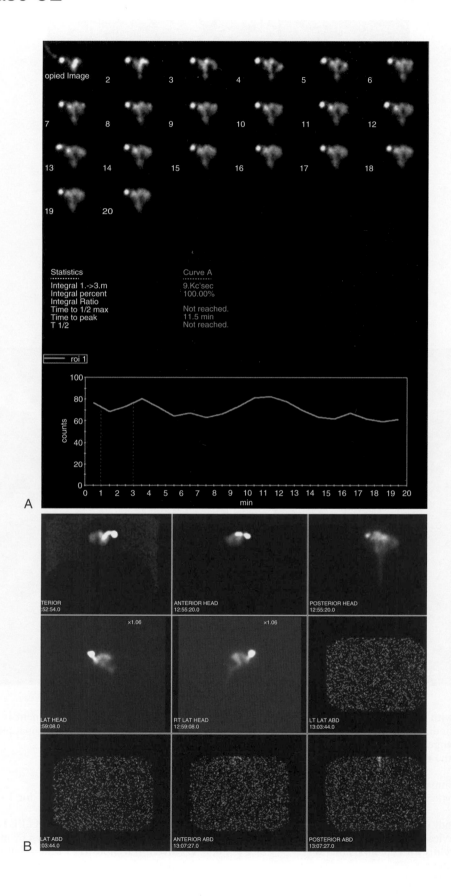

1. What is the likeliest clinical history that would prompt this study?
   a. Dysphagia
   b. Headaches
   c. Pain
   d. Extremity numbness
2. What is the radiopharmaceutical most likely to be utilized?
   a. Tc-99m DTPA
   b. Tc-99m RBC
   c. Tc-99m SC
   d. In-111 WBC
3. What is the expected half-time for a normal study?
   a. Less than 10 minutes
   b. 10–20 minutes
   c. 20–30 minutes
   d. Greater than 30 minutes
4. What is the likely diagnosis if the system empties after ambulation?
   a. Normal
   b. Positional obstruction
   c. Patulous system
   d. Complete obstruction

Case 93

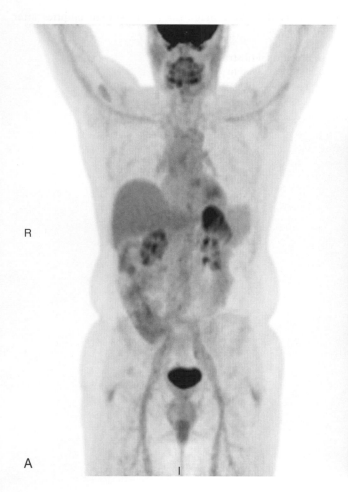

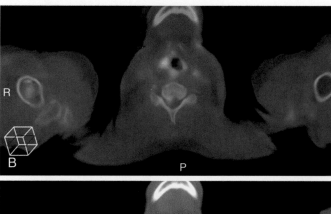

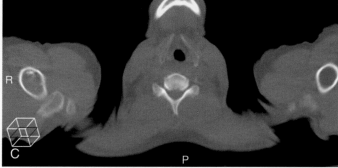

Images from an F-18 FDG PET/CT scan in a patient who is in remission from lymphoma are shown.

1. Where is the abnormality located?
   a. Left humerus
   b. Right humerus
   c. Glenoid
   d. Thoracic spine

2. All of the following benign bone lesions may typically show low-grade FDG uptake EXCEPT:
   a. Hemangioma
   b. Enchondroma
   c. Intraosseous lipoma
   d. Giant cell tumor

3. All of the following are CT characteristics of an aggressive osseous lesion EXCEPT:
   a. Wide zone of transition
   b. Onion-skin periosteal reaction
   c. Thick sclerotic margin
   d. Cortical breakthrough with an associated soft tissue mass

4. Which of the following best describes a benign enchondroma?
   a. Proximal metaphyseal lesion with chondroid matrix (rings and arcs), no endosteal scalloping or sclerotic margin
   b. Diaphyseal lesion with well-defined sclerotic margin and ground-glass central matrix
   c. Proximal metaphyseal lesion with chondroid matrix, deep endosteal scalloping, and endosteal cortical thickening
   d. Cartilage-capped osseous excrescence, with continuous cortex and marrow extending from underlying bone

Case 94

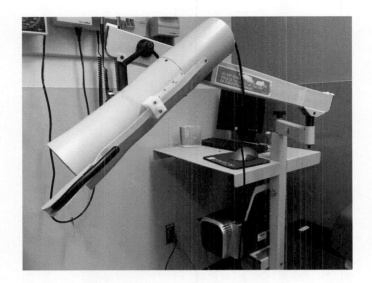

1. What is the equipment shown in the image?
   a. Well counter
   b. Geiger counter
   c. Thyroid probe
   d. Dose calibrator
2. What is the primary photopeak for I-123?
   a. 81 keV
   b. 140 keV
   c. 159 keV
   d. 247 keV
3. What is the mode of decay for I-123?
   a. Positron emission
   b. Beta emission
   c. Electron capture
   d. Isomeric transition
4. Why should this instrument be placed at a close, fixed distance from the patient?
   a. For consistency
   b. To eliminate extraneous radiation
   c. To reduce the amount of radiation to the patient
   d. A and B

Case 95

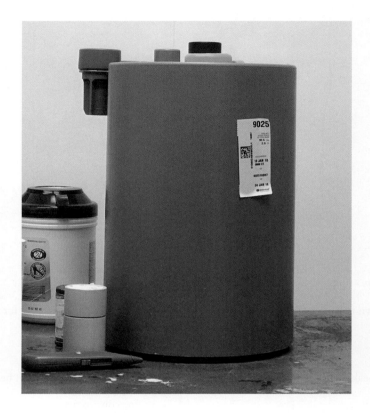

1. In a Mo-99 generator, the maximum buildup of Tc-99m occurs how many hours after the last elution?
   a. 6
   b. 12
   c. 16
   d. 23
2. What is the half-life of Mo-99?
   a. 24 hours
   b. 1.7 days
   c. 2.8 days
   d. 3.8 days
3. What is the Nuclear Regulatory Commission (NRC) limit of Mo-99 activity per 2 mCi of Tc-99m in an administered dose?
   a. 0.15 μCi
   b. 0.3 μCi
   c. 0.15 mCi
   d. 0.3 mCi
4. Evaluation for the presence of aluminum oxide (Al_2O_3) in the eluate measures:
   a. Radionuclide purity
   b. Chemical purity
   c. Radiochemical purity
   d. Pyrogenicity

Case 96

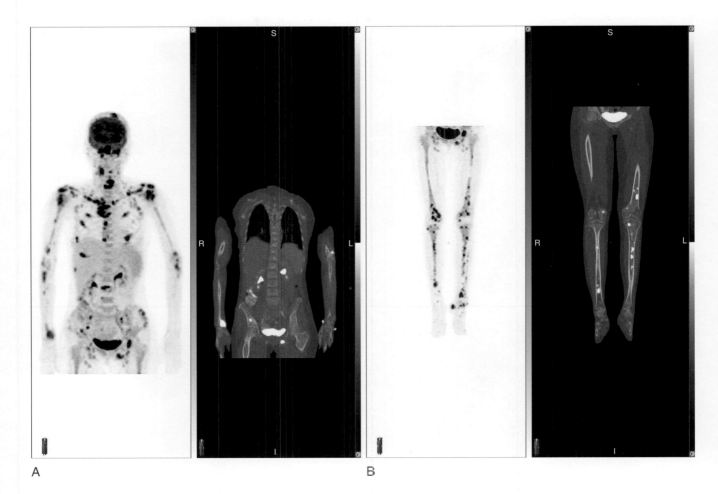

A   B

A 34-year-old female, who is a recent immigrant from Vietnam, presented with fatigue, general malaise, and numerous osseous lesions detected on CT and was referred for a whole-body PET/CT scan. Images showed numerous hypermetabolic mixed lytic and sclerotic lesions in the axial and appendicular skeleton. There was no hypermetabolic solid organ involvement.

1. All of the following are included in the differential EXCEPT:
   a. Metastatic disease
   b. Multiple myeloma
   c. Disseminated osteomyelitis
   d. Multiple hereditary exostosis
2. Which cells contribute to FDG uptake in infection/inflammation?
   a. Macrophages
   b. Neutrophils
   c. Lymphocytes
   d. All of the above

3. What is the mechanism of increased FDG uptake in inflammatory cells and tumor cells?
   a. Upregulation of insulin-like growth factor 1 (IGF-1) and IGF-2
   b. Upregulation of glucose transporter 1 (GLUT1)
   c. Increased affinity for deoxyglucose caused by cytokines
   d. Upregulation of GLUT2 and GLUT15
4. Which of the following is a major indications for 18F FDG PET/CT in infection and inflammation?
   a. Sarcoidosis
   b. Peripheral bone osteomyelitis
   c. Evaluation of fever of unknown origin (FUO)
   d. All of the above

Case 97

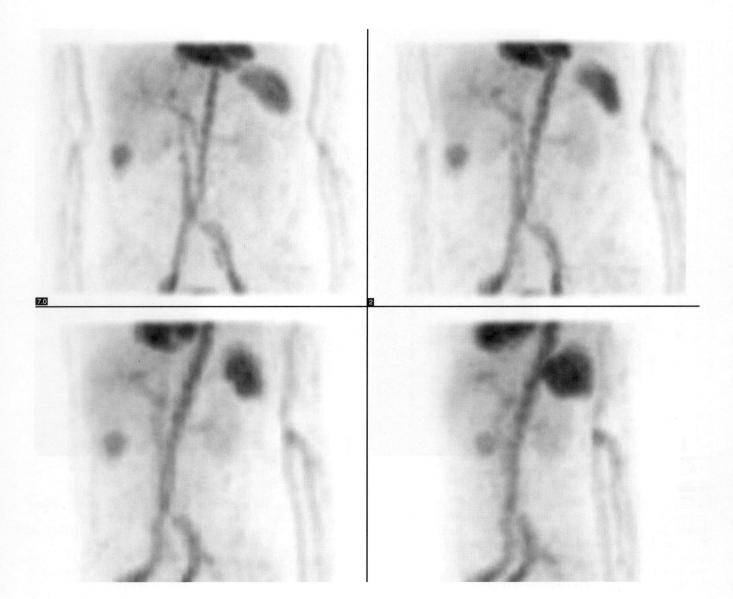

1. What is the salient finding?
   a. Common bile duct (CBD) obstruction
   b. Cystic duct obstruction
   c. Liver lesion
   d. Liver dysfunction
2. What is the radiopharmaceutical?
   a. Tc-99m mebrofenin
   b. Tc-99m RBC
   c. Tc-99m MDP
   d. Tc-99 DTPA
3. What is the diagnosis?
   a. Hemangioma
   b. Metastases
   c. Acute cholecystitis
   d. Hepatitis
4. What is the most likely etiology for a false-negative result?
   a. Site of primary malignancy
   b. Histology of primary malignancy
   c. Size of lesion
   d. Liver function

Case 98

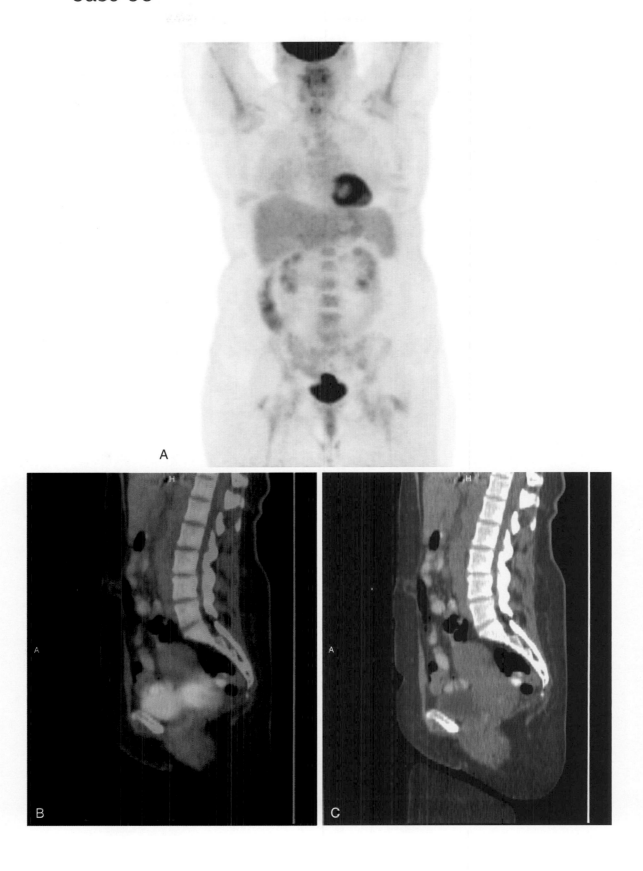

A

B

C

Multiple images from an F-18 FDG PET/CT scan in a patient with recently diagnosed cervical cancer are shown.

1. Which of the following statements best describes the role of PET/CT in the management of cervical cancer?
   a. PET/CT is the modality of choice for determination of extent of primary tumor and is superior to MRI and CT.
   b. PET/CT is the modality of choice for initial staging and management of recurrent disease.
   c. PET/CT is recommended annually for surveillance in asymptomatic patients after treatment.
   d. PET/CT is superior to MRI in the evaluating parametrial spread of tumor.

2. What is the major risk factor for cervical cancer?
   a. History of sexually transmitted diseases (STDs)
   b. Cigarette smoking
   c. Infection with human papilloma virus (HPV)
   d. Early onset of sexual activity

3. In this case, there is focal uptake in the cervix (SUV_{max} 11) corresponding to the hypoenhancing mass on the MRI scan. No regional hypermetabolic nodes or distant metastatic disease is present on the MIP. What is the tumor staging?
   a. Stage I
   b. Stage II
   c. Stage III
   d. Stage IV

4. Physiologic urinary bladder activity may obscure the primary tumor and confound interpretation of local lymph nodes. Which technique would mitigate this problem?
   a. Urinary bladder catheterization
   b. Administration of diuretics and oral hydration
   c. Repeat imaging of the pelvis after voiding
   d. All of the above

Case 99

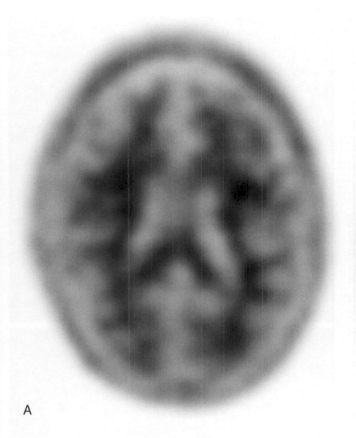

A

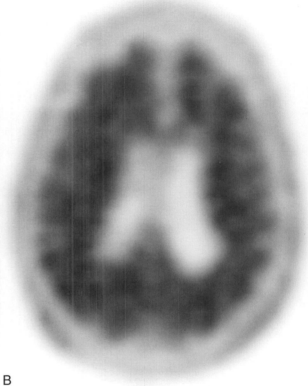

B

1. Which radiopharmaceutical is approved by the U.S. Food and Drug Administration (FDA) for detection of amyloid plaques in the brain?
   a. F-18 FDG PET
   b. Tc-99m HMPAO
   c. F-18 florbetapir
   d. Carbon-11 (C-11) Pittsburg compound B (PiB)
2. The target for this radiopharmaceutical is found in which of the following locations?
   a. Between neurons
   b. Within neurons
   c. Dendrites
   d. Astrocytes

3. In what setting is radiolabeled amyloid imaging appropriate?
   a. Patients with core clinical criteria for probable Alzheimer's disease
   b. Assessment of the severity of dementia
   c. Persistent or progressive unexplained mild cognitive impairment (MCI)
   d. Asymptomatic patients wishing to know their possible future risk
4. What patient preparation is recommended before study initiation?
   a. NPO for 6 hours before injection
   b. Restrict long-acting insulin for 12 hours before injection
   c. No patient preparation
   d. High-fat diet for 12 hours before injection

Case 100

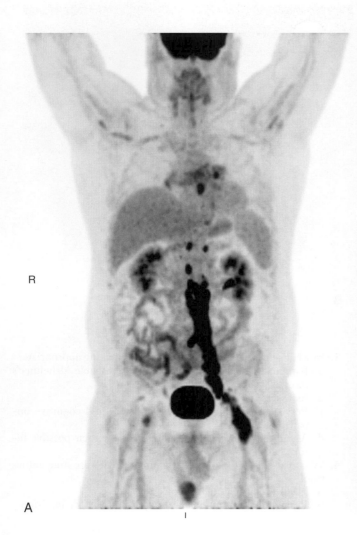

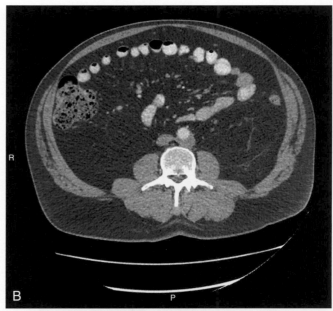

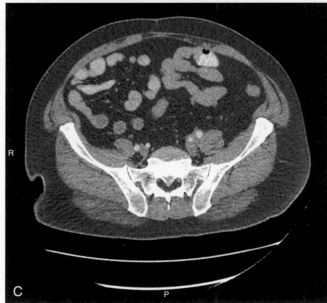

1. What is the likely diagnosis?
   a. Thrombus
   b. Lymphatic obstruction
   c. Retroperitoneal fibrosis
   d. Atherosclerotic disease
2. How may this entity be treated?
   a. Immunosuppressive therapy
   b. Tamoxifen
   c. Surgery
   d. All of the above

3. Which adjacent structure(s) are most commonly affected?
   a. Pancreas
   b. Bladder
   c. Adrenal glands
   d. Ureters
4. What is the next step in the management of this patient?
   a. Magnetic resonance angiography (MRA) of the aorta and iliac vessels
   b. Diagnostic angiography
   c. Biopsy
   d. Surgery

Case 101

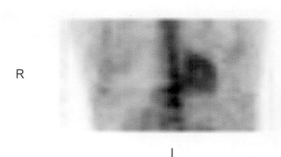

Image A

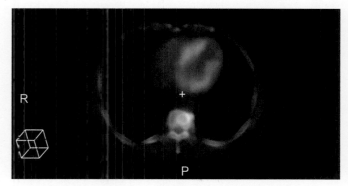

Image B

1. The gold standard for diagnosing cardiac amyloid is:
   a. Magnetic resonance imaging (MRI)
   b. Endocardial biopsy
   c. Myocardial perfusion study
   d. Echocardiography
2. What radiopharmaceutical may be utilized for the diagnosis of cardiac amyloidosis?
   a. Technetium-99m (Tc-99m) mercaptoacetyltriglycine (MAG3)
   b. Tc-99m diethylene-triamine-penta-acetate (DTPA)
   c. Tc-99m pyrophosphate (PYP)
   d. Tc-99m sestamibi

3. Which type of cardiac amyloidosis may be diagnosed with the above radiopharmaceutical?
   a. Immunoglobulin light-chain amyloidosis
   b. Transthyretin-related cardiac amyloidosis
   c. Neurofibrillary tangles
   d. All subtypes
4. What is the histopathology of cardiac amyloidosis?
   a. Intracellular deposition of fibrillary protein
   b. Intracellular neurofibrillary tangles
   c. Extracellular deposition of fibrillary protein
   d. Binding to mitochondria

Case 102

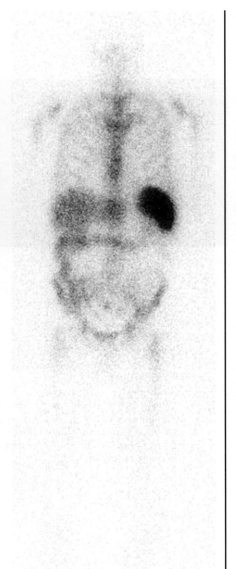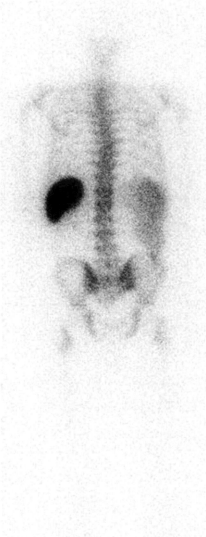

1. What is the radiopharmaceutical?
   a. Indium-111 (In-111) leukocytes
   b. In-111 pentetreotide
   c. I-123 metaiodobenzylguanidine (MIBG)
   d. Tc-99m methylene diphosphonate (MDP)
2. What is the abnormality?
   a. Uptake in the kidneys
   b. Uptake in the proximal large bowel
   c. Increased uptake in the spleen relative to the liver
   d. Uptake in bone marrow

3. What is the most likely diagnosis?
   a. Pyelonephritis
   b. Splenic abscess
   c. Osteomyelitis
   d. Colitis
4. Standard imaging occurs at:
   a. 2 hours
   b. 12 hours
   c. 24 hours
   d. 48 hours

Case 103

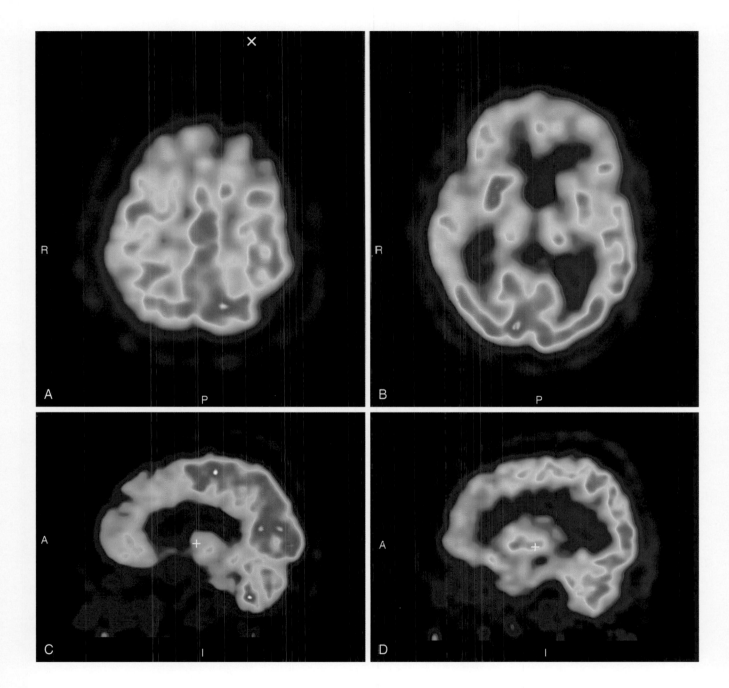

1. What is the salient finding on this fluorine-18 fluorodeoxyglu-cose (F-18 FDG) brain scan?
   a. Hypometabolism primarily involving the frontal lobes
   b. Hypometabolism primarily involving the parietal lobes
   c. Focal increased FDG avidity in the left parietal lobe suspicious for underlying neoplasia
   d. Focal increased FDG avidity in the left frontal lobe suspicious for underlying neoplasia
2. What is the most likely diagnosis?
   a. Alzheimer's disease
   b. Pick's disease
   c. Lewy body disease dementia
   d. Primary progressive aphasia
3. The pathologic correlate for this disease is best characterized as:
   a. Tauopathy
   b. Amyloid plaque deposition
   c. Somatostatin receptor positive tissue
   d. Gliosis
4. What other radiopharmaceutical may be considered for the evaluation of this patient's disease?
   a. Tc-99m HMPAO
   b. Tc-99m DTPA
   c. F-18 florbetapir
   d. Tc-99m sestamibi

Case 104

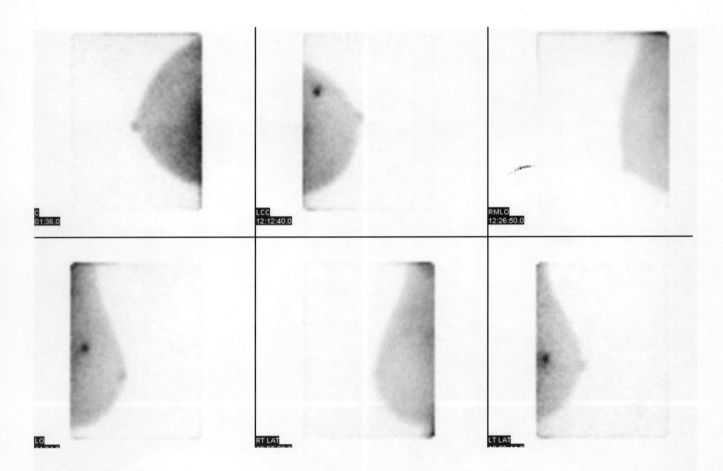

1. What is the study radiotracer?
   a. Tc-99m DTPA
   b. Tc-99m sestamibi
   c. Tc-99m MAG3
   d. Tc-99m tilmanocept
2. What is the mechanism of uptake?
   a. Phosphorylated and trapped within the cell
   b. Concentrated in mitochondria as a function of charge
   c. Adsorption to hydroxyapatite
   d. Secreted in the proximal tubules

3. Which entity demonstrates focal uptake with Tc-99m sestamibi?
   a. Ductal carcinoma in situ
   b. Invasive ductal carcinoma
   c. Fibroadenoma
   d. All of the above
4. What may cause a false-positive result?
   a. Does not occur
   b. Nothing by mouth (NPO) 4 hours before examination not done by patient
   c. Fine needle aspiration (FNA) breast biopsy 1 week before examination
   d. Recent administration of long-acting insulin

Case 105

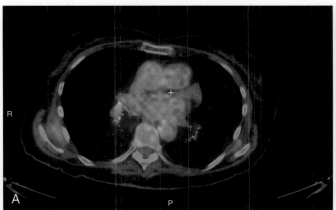 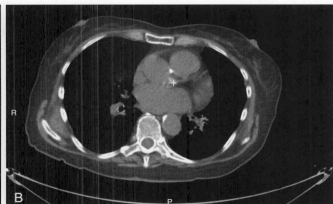

1. What is the salient finding on this F18 FDG positron-emission tomography/computed tomography (PET/CT) performed for the evaluation of a fever of unknown origin?
   a. FDG-avid focus at the inferior aspect of the right scapula
   b. FDG-avid focus in the sternum
   c. Physiologic muscular activity adjacent to the right scapula
   d. FDG-avid pulmonary nodule concerning for malignancy
2. What is the most likely diagnosis?
   a. Physiologic muscle activity
   b. Metastases
   c. Lipoma
   d. Elastofibroma dorsi

3. What is the indicated management?
   a. No intervention or follow-up needed
   b. Radiation
   c. Chemotherapy
   d. Biopsy
4. What is the most likely patient demographic for this finding?
   a. 20-year-old female
   b. 20-year-old male
   c. 65-year-old female
   d. 65-year-old male

Case 106

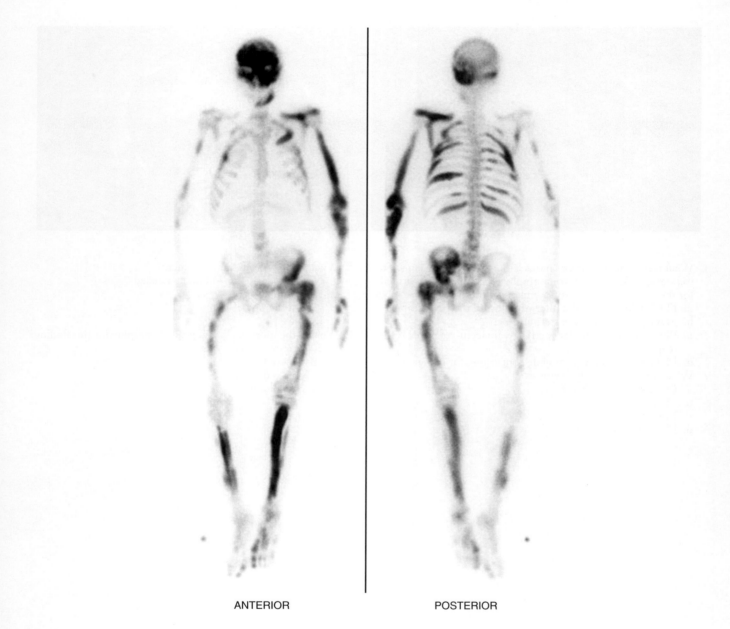

ANTERIOR   POSTERIOR

1. What is the most likely diagnosis?
    a. Polyostotic fibrous dysplasia
    b. Osseous metastases
    c. Osteomyelitis
    d. Osteochondromas
2. What is the main etiology for the osseous abnormality?
    a. Increased osteoclast activity
    b. Increased fibroblast activity
    c. Increased osteoblast activity
    d. Increase in cancellous bone

3. What may be noted on physical examination?
    a. Café au lait spots
    b. Hemangiomas
    c. Atypical nevi
    d. Dermatofibromas
4. If the patient has precocious puberty and bone pain, what syndrome should be considered?
    a. Zollinger-Ellison syndrome
    b. Maffucci's syndrome
    c. Ollier's syndrome
    d. McCune-Albright syndrome

Case 107

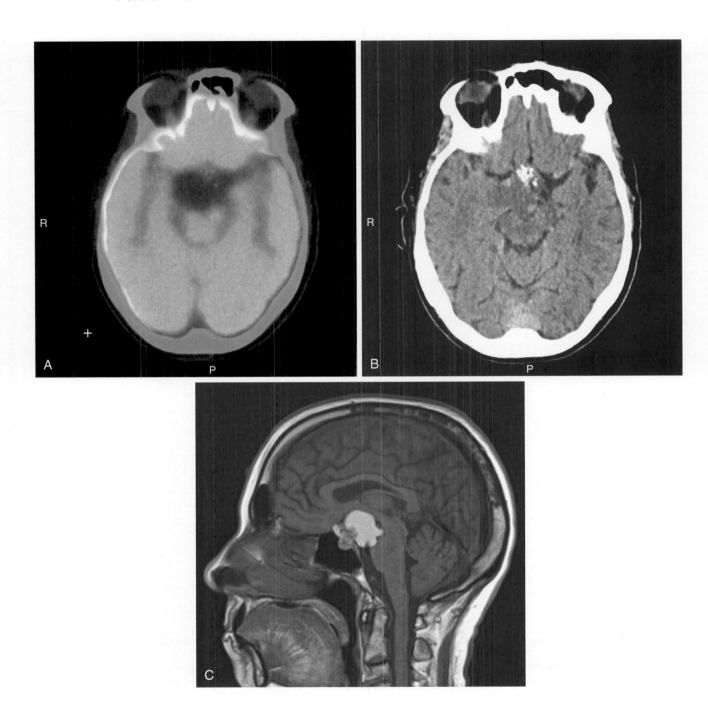

1. What is the salient finding on this F-18 FDG PET scan?
   a. Focal area of increased uptake in the region of the sella
   b. Focal area of decreased uptake in the region of the sella
   c. Focal increase uptake in the left frontal white matter
   d. Reduced cortical uptake in the left frontal lobe
2. Correlating this study with the CT study, what is your interpretation?
   a. Metastatic lesion
   b. Glioblastoma
   c. Craniopharyngioma
   d. Lymphoma
3. Which statement best describes the incidence in the patient population with this tumor?
   a. Occurs primarily in children less than 10 years of age
   b. Occurs primarily in adults greater than 50 years of age
   c. Bimodal distribution with peaks in the early teens and adults over age 50 years
   d. No definitive trends in age distribution
4. These tumors tend to occur in the:
   a. Sellar/suprasellar regions
   b. Temporal lobes
   c. Frontal lobes
   d. Posterior fossa

Case 108

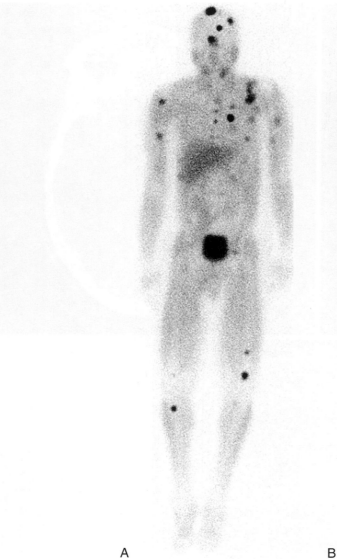

A

B

1. What is the likely diagnosis on this I-123 MIBG scan?
   a. Metastatic breast cancer
   b. Metastatic pheochromocytoma/paraganglioma
   c. Polyostotic fibrous dysplasia
   d. Multiple hereditary exostosis
2. What receptor does the radiopharmaceutical target?
   a. Somatostatin
   b. Vascular endothelial growth factor (VEGF)
   c. Norepinephrine
   d. Prostate-specific membrane antigen (PSMA)

3. All of the following characteristics increase the risk of metastatic disease EXCEPT:
   a. Large size of primary lesion
   b. Primary lesion outside the adrenal gland (paraganglioma)
   c. Primary lesion in the adrenal gland (pheochromocytoma)
   d. Succinyl dehydrogenase enzyme deficiency
4. Which one of the following nuclear medicine therapies may be considered for treatment?
   a. I-131 MIBG
   b. I 131
   c. Yttrium-90 (Y-90) microspheres
   d. Lu-177 PSMA

Case 109

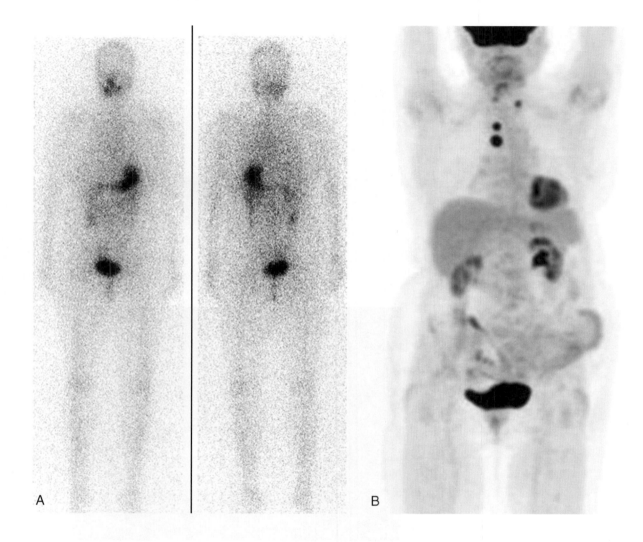

A

B

1. What is the finding on image A?
   a. I-123 scan without evidence of metastatic disease
   b. I-123 scan with evidence of metastatic disease in the bowel
   c. I-123 scan with residual disease in the thyroid bed
   d. I-123 scan with cervical adenopathy
2. What is the next step in the radiologic evaluation of a patient with elevated serum thyroglobulin?
   a. No imaging indicated
   b. F-18 FDG PET/CT
   c. F18 fluciclovine
   d. I-131 whole-body imaging

3. What is the likely histologic explanation for the findings on Image B?
   a. No residual thyroid cancer
   b. Focal infection in the lower neck
   c. Residual thyroid cancer that has transformed into a higher-grade poorly differentiated tumor
   d. Residual thyroid cancer that has transformed into a lower-grade tumor
4. What is the next step in the management of this patient?
   a. Repeat I-131 therapy (high dose)
   b. Repeat I-131 therapy (low dose)
   c. Surgical resection of nodal disease
   d. Total thyroidectomy

Case 110

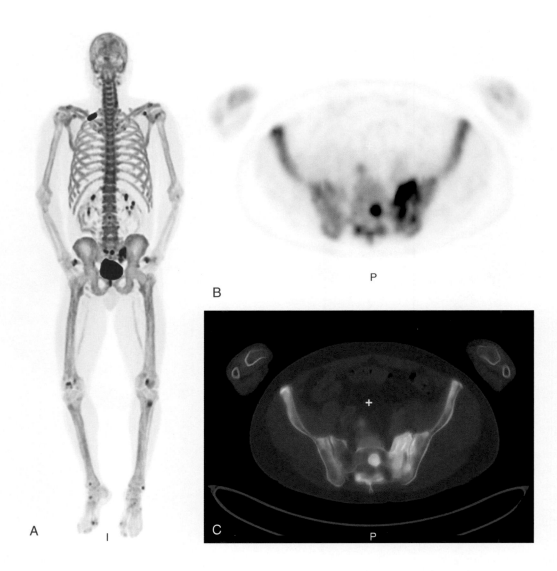

A

B

P

C

P

I

1. What is the PET radiotracer?
   a. F-18 FDG
   b. F-18 sodium fluoride (NaF)
   c. Ga-68 DOTA-TATE
   d. F-18 fluciclovine (FACBC)
2. What is the most likely indication for this study?
   a. Neurodegenerative disease
   b. Osseous metastases
   c. Granulomatous disease
   d. Neuroendocrine tumor evaluation
3. Which study has the highest specificity for the evaluation for osseous metastases?
   a. Tc-99m MDP planar whole-body imaging
   b. F-18 NaF PET
   c. F-18 NaF PET/CT
   d. Tc-99m SPECT MDP
4. The mode of decay for F-18 sodium fluoride (NaF) is:
   a. Alpha emission
   b. Positron emission
   c. Beta decay
   d. Electron capture

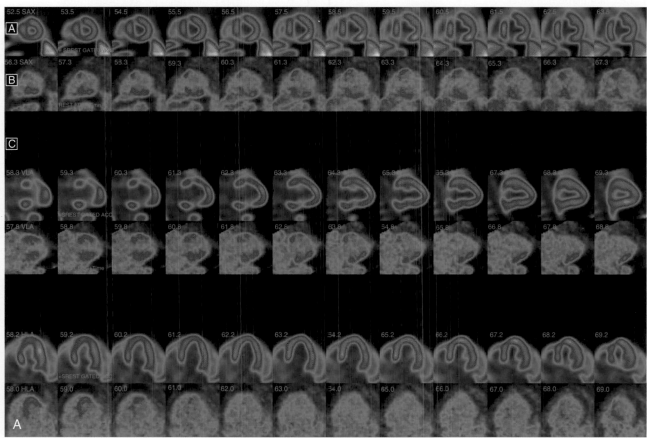

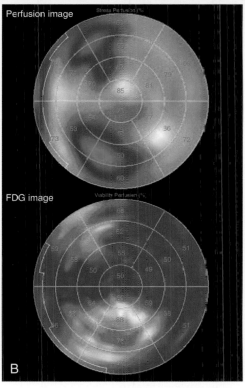

1. In a patient with history of granulomatous disease, what is the most likely diagnosis?
    a. Cardiac sarcoidosis
    b. Myocardial infarction
    c. Cardiac ischemia
    d. Left bundle branch block
2. Which tracer may be used to perform perfusion PET imaging?
    a. F-18 FDG
    b. Nitrogen-13 (NH-13) ammonia
    c. Tc-99m sestamibi
    d. F-18 florbetapir
3. Which tracer is used to evaluate for underlying inflammation?
    a. F-18 FDG
    b. NH-13 ammonia
    c. Tc-99m sestamibi
    d. F-18 florbetapir
4. What is the recommended patient preparation?
    a. None
    b. NPO for 4 hours before examination
    c. High-fat, low-carbohydrate diet before radiopharmaceutical injection
    d. High-carbohydrate, low-fat diet before radiopharmaceutical injection

Case 112

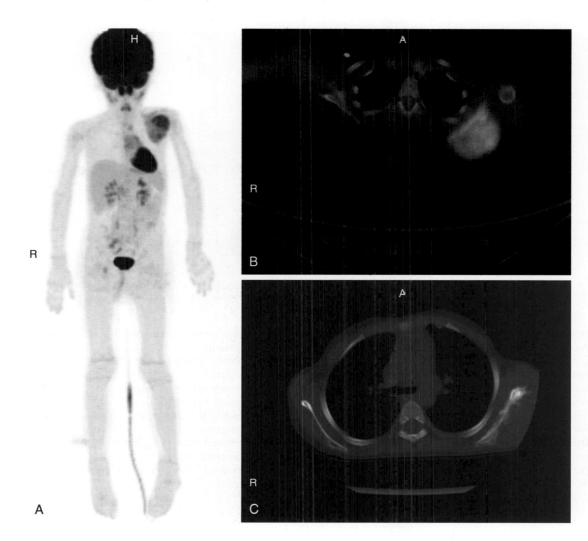

1. What is the salient finding?
   a. Physiologic muscular activity related to recent exercise
   b. Aggressive-appearing FDG-avid lesion centered on the left scapula
   c. Benign-appearing FDG-avid lesion centered on the left scapula
   d. Abnormal FDG activity centered on the left scapula, likely related to recent trauma
2. What is the most likely diagnosis?
   a. Neuroblastoma
   b. Ewing's sarcoma
   c. Osteomyelitis
   d. Congenital deformity

3. What age group is most likely to be diagnosed with this entity?
   a. Less than 1 years
   b. 5–25 years
   c. 26–50 years
   d. Greater than 50 years
4. The most likely site of primary disease is:
   a. Femur
   b. Spine
   c. Pelvis
   d. Skull

Case 113

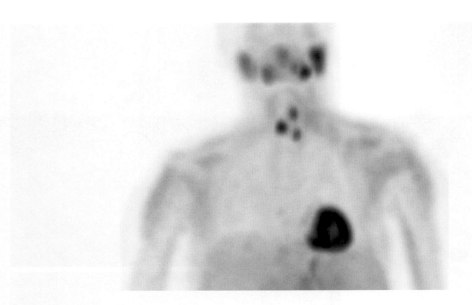

The patient has renal failure and elevated serum calcium, and this Tc-99m sestamibi scan was obtained.

1. What is your interpretation of the study?
   a. Metastatic thyroid cancer
   b. Primary hyperparathyroidism
   c. Secondary hyperparathyroidism
   d. Tertiary hyperparathyroidism
2. The most common cause for secondary hyperparathyroidism is:
   a. Malignancy
   b. Chronic renal failure
   c. Hyperthyroidism
   d. Paget's disease
3. Untreated or poorly responsive secondary hyperparathyroidism may result in:
   a. Primary hyperparathyroidism
   b. Tertiary hyperparathyroidism
   c. Primary hyperthyroidism
   d. Primary hypothyroidism
4. The underlying etiology for secondary hyperparathyroidism is:
   a. Decreased active vitamin D levels
   b. Increased vitamin B_{12} levels
   c. Decreased vitamin B_{12} levels
   d. Increased active vitamin D levels

Case 114

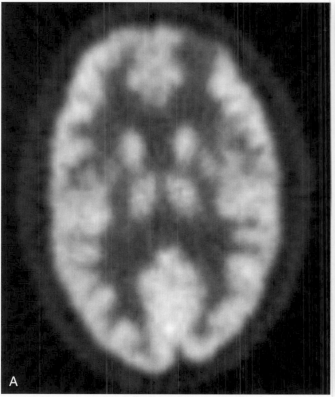 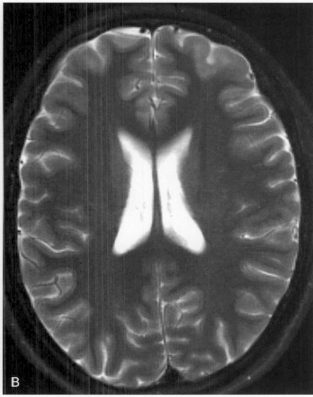

1. What is the salient finding of this F-18 FDG PET brain study?
   a. Focal decreased uptake in the left frontal lobe
   b. Focal decreased uptake in the right frontal lobe
   c. Increased metabolic uptake in the basal ganglia
   d. Focal increased uptake in the left frontal white matter
2. Of the following choices, what is the most likely etiology?
   a. Abscess
   b. Encephalitis
   c. Pachymeningitis
   d. Seizure focus
3. What is the next step?
   a. Magnetic resonance imaging (MRI) of the brain
   b. Cerebrospinal fluid (CSF) analysis
   c. CT myelography
   d. In-111 DTPA CSF flow study
4. All of the following can present as focal cortical decreased uptake EXCEPT:
   a. Interictal seizure focus
   b. Low-grade malignancy
   c. Infarct
   d. Physiologic cortical activity

Case 115

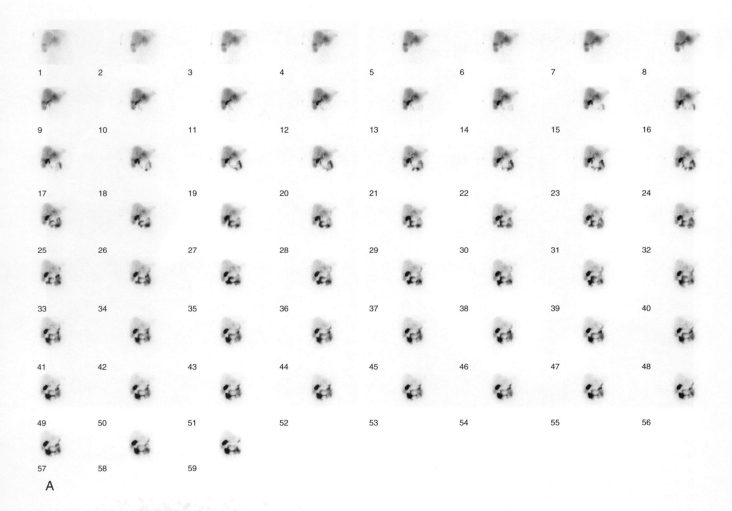

1   2   3   4   5   6   7   8

9   10   11   12   13   14   15   16

17   18   19   20   21   22   23   24

25   26   27   28   29   30   31   32

33   34   35   36   37   38   39   40

41   42   43   44   45   46   47   48

49   50   51   52   53   54   55   56

57   58   59

A

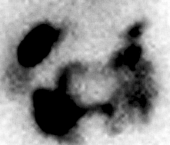

B

1. What radiotracer was utilized?
   a. Tc-99m MDP
   b. Tc-99m DTPA
   c. Tc-99m mebrofenin
   d. Tc-99m MAG3
2. What is the finding?
   a. Rim's sign
   b. Focal increased hepatic uptake
   c. Enterogastric reflux
   d. Biliary leak
3. The patient is a 25-year-old female with no history of chronic liver disease or malignancy. What is the likely diagnosis?
   a. Focal segmental intrahepatic biliary obstruction
   b. Hepatoma
   c. Focal nodular hyperplasia (FNH)
   d. Hepatic adenoma
4. What other radiopharmaceutical can help make this diagnosis with some certainty?
   a. Tc-99m sulfur colloid (SC)
   b. In-111 Octreoscan
   c. Tc-99m MDP
   d. Tc-99m hexamethylpropyleneamine oxime (HMPAO)

Case 116

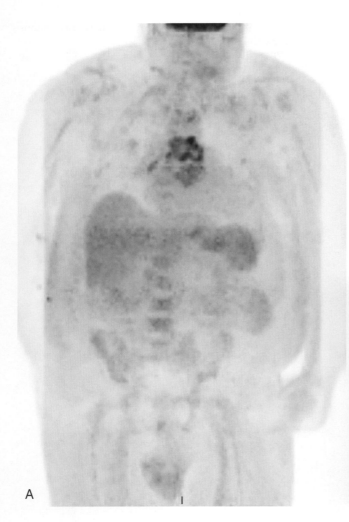

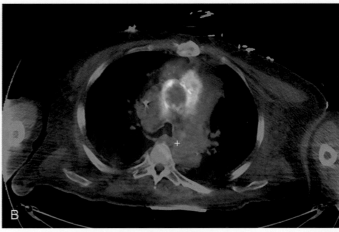

1. What is the salient finding on this F-18 FDG PET study?
   a. Abnormal radiotracer activity in the region of the aortic valve
   b. Abnormal radiotracer activity at the apex of the left ventricle
   c. Abnormal radiotracer activity involving the pericardium
   d. Normal physiologic activity
2. What is the most likely etiology for this in a patient with bacteremia?
   a. Endocarditis
   b. Myxofibroma
   c. Myocardial infarction
   d. Physiologic activity

3. What is the most likely next step in the workup of this patient?
   a. No additional workup needed
   b. Transesophageal echocardiography (TEE)
   c. Surgery
   d. Cardiac catheterization
4. What additional scintigraphic study may be of value in the setting of endocarditis?
   a. In-111 white blood cell (WBC) scan
   b. Tc-99m MDP bone scan
   c. Tc-99 SC scan
   d. Tc-99m dimercaptosuccinic acid (DMSA) scan

Case 117

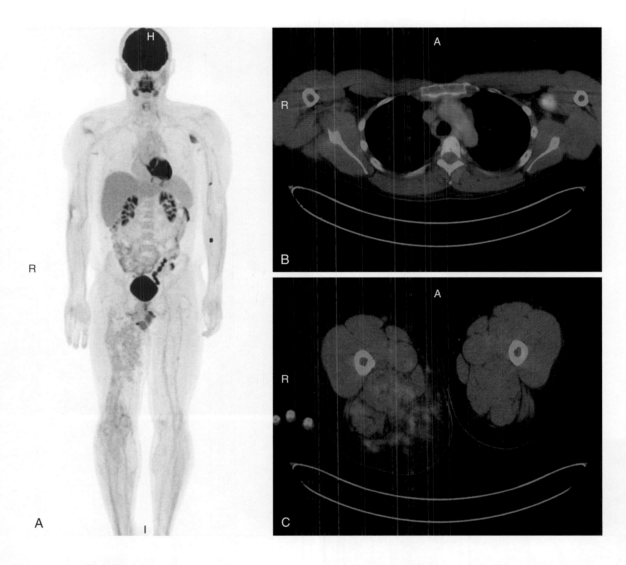

1. What is the most likely diagnosis on this F-18 FDG PET/CT scan?
   a. Physiologic activity
   b. Infiltration of radiotracer
   c. Plexiform neurofibromas
   d. Contusion
2. Why is an FDG PET/CT performed in this patient population?
   a. To determine how many lesions there are
   b. To determine whether these lesions have undergone malignant transformation
   c. To evaluate for locoregional disease
   d. To assess for myositis
3. What is the likely underlying disease?
   a. Sarcoidosis
   b. Diabetes mellitus
   c. Neurofibromatosis
   d. Zollinger-Ellison syndrome
4. All of the following may be identified on clinical examination as manifestations of this disease EXCEPT:
   a. Lisch's nodules
   b. Café au lait spots
   c. Cutaneous neurofibromas
   d. Acanthosis nigricans

Case 118

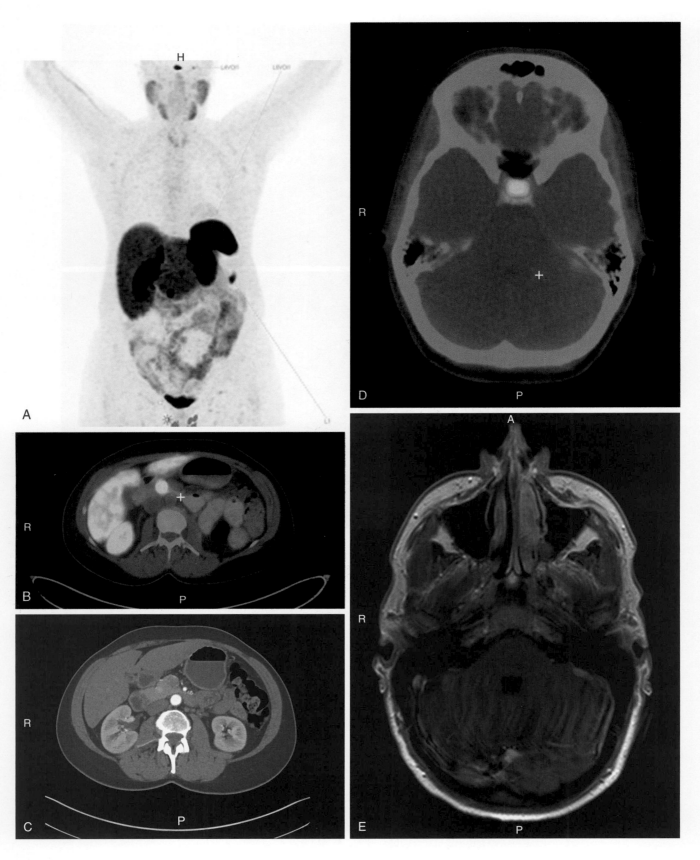

1. What is the half-life of the radionuclide Ga-68?
   a. 6 minutes
   b. 13 minutes
   c. 68 minutes
   d. 78 minutes
2. What is the radiopharmaceutical?
   a. Ga-68 DOTA-TATE
   b. Ga-67 citrate
   c. I-131
   d. F-18 FDG
3. Physiologic uptake may be seen with this radiopharmaceutical in all of the following sites EXCEPT:
   a. Adrenal glands
   b. Spleen
   c. Heart
   d. Kidneys
4. What is the mechanism of uptake of this radiopharmaceutical?
   a. Amino acid metabolism
   b. Norepinephrine analog
   c. Somatostatin receptor
   d. PSMA

Case 119

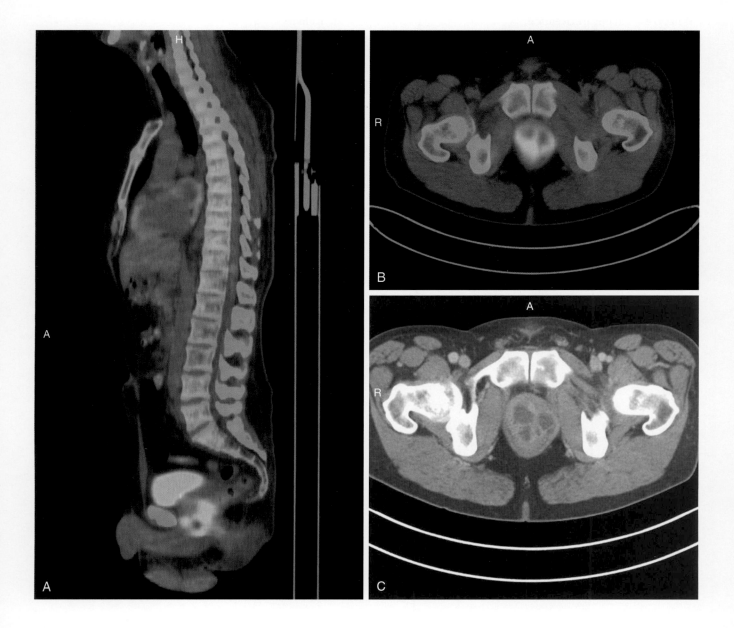

1. What is the salient finding?
   a. Urine contamination
   b. Physiologic activity
   c. Abnormal radiotracer activity in the prostate
   d. Bladder diverticulum

2. What is the most likely etiology based on the CT findings?
   a. Prostate cancer
   b. Prostate abscess
   c. Rectal carcinoma
   d. Pelvic adenopathy

3. What is the most likely cause for prostate abscesses?
   a. Prostatitis
   b. Prostate cancer
   c. Radiation therapy
   d. Direct extension from bowel wall infection/inflammation

4. Classic CT findings of prostatic abscesses include:
   a. Hypodense lesions in an enlarged gland
   b. Periprostatic inflammatory changes in a shrunken gland
   c. Uniform enhancement in the prostate gland
   d. No definitive CT findings.

Case 120

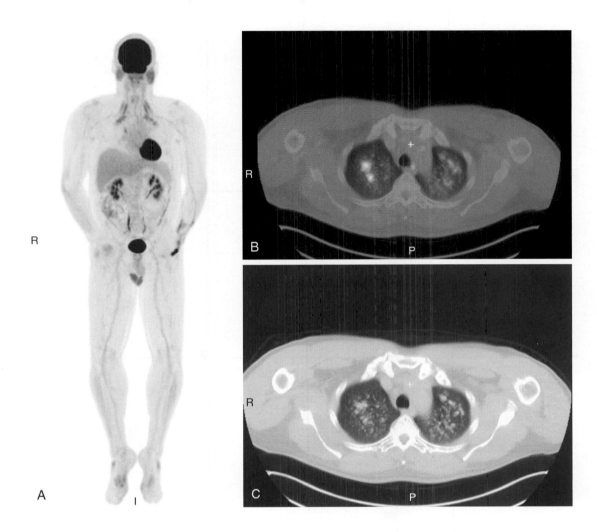

1. What is the salient finding in this patient with a history of multiple myeloma?
   a. Hypermetabolic supraclavicular adenopathy
   b. Hypermetabolic rib lesions
   c. Hypermetabolic fluffy, apical lung nodules
   d. Hypermetabolic lung masses
2. What is the most likely diagnosis?
   a. Metastatic disease from osteosarcoma
   b. Pulmonary infarcts
   c. Metastatic pulmonary calcifications
   d. Granulomatous disease

3. All of the following conditions may result in metastatic pulmonary calcifications EXCEPT:
   a. Chronic renal failure
   b. Multiple myeloma
   c. Hyperparathyroidism
   d. Hyperthyroidism
4. The most likely pathophysiologic explanation for this finding is:
   a. More alkaline environment in the lung apices
   b. Increased perfusion to ventilation ratio in the lung apices
   c. More acidic environment in the lung apices
   d. Increased ventilation to perfusion ratio at the lung bases

Case 121

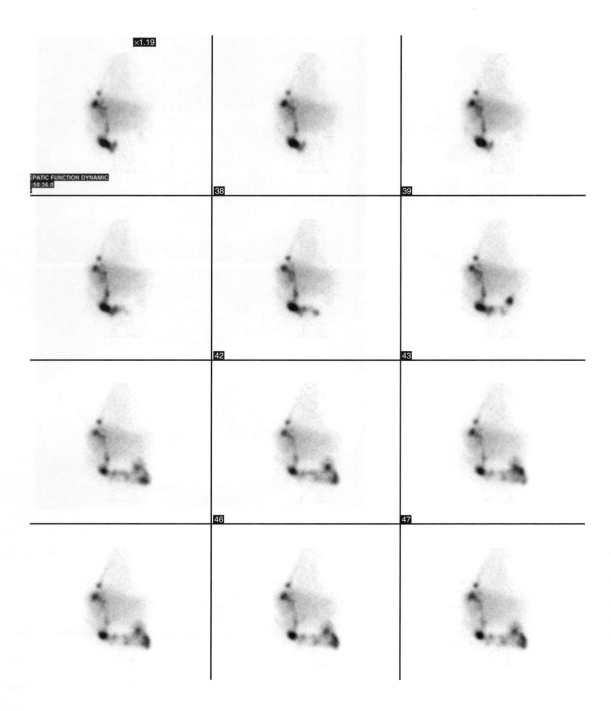

1. What is the radiopharmaceutical?
   a. Tc-99m mebrofenin
   b. Tc-99m MDP
   c. Tc-99m MAG3
   d. Tc-99m DTPA
2. What is the diagnosis?
   a. Hepatobronchial fistula
   b. Bile leak
   c. Diaphragmatic rupture
   d. Bronchopleural fistula

3. Likely etiologies include all of the following EXCEPT:
   a. Congenital anomaly
   b. Hepatic or subdiaphragmatic abscess
   c. Focal nodular hyperplasia
   d. Hepatic tumor
4. How would the technique change if the patient had hyperbilirubinemia?
   a. Increase the radiopharmaceutical dose
   b. Decrease the radiopharmaceutical dose
   c. No change indicated
   d. Cannot perform the study

Case 122

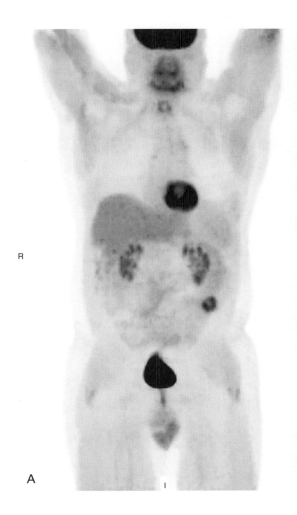

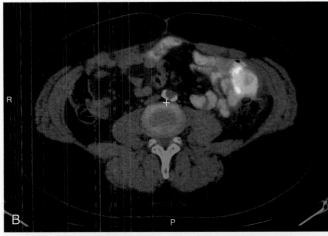

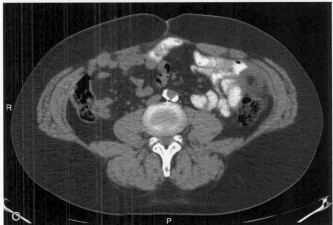

1. Describe the salient finding.
   a. FDG-avid bowel lesion suspicious for primary malignancy
   b. Physiologic bowel activity
   c. FDG-avid density with central fat outside the bowel lumen
   d. Physiologic renal activity
2. What is the most likely diagnosis?
   a. Colon cancer
   b. Fat necrosis
   c. Peritoneal metastases
   d. Lymphadenopathy

3. Epiploic appendages are most commonly located in which area?
   a. Left colon
   b. Right colon
   c. Small bowel
   d. Rectum
4. What is the best treatment plan for epiploic appendagitis?
   a. Surgery
   b. Radiation
   c. Chemotherapy
   d. Supportive care as epiploic appendagitis is self-limiting

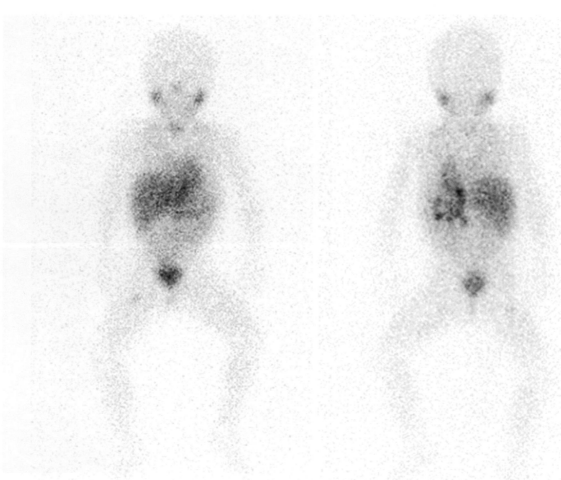

A   B

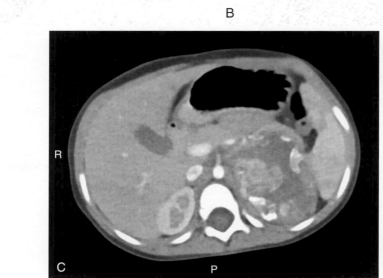

1. What is the radiopharmaceutical?
   a. I-123 MIBG
   b. F18 FDG PET/CT
   c. In-111 Octreoscan (pentetreotide)
   d. In-111 WBC
2. What is the most likely diagnosis?
   a. Metastatic pheochromocytoma
   b. Metastatic neuroblastoma
   c. Metastatic renal cell cancer
   d. Metastatic carcinoid
3. Most of these tumors originate in the:
   a. Chest
   b. Retroperitoneal region
   c. Extremities
   d. Periorbital region
4. The highest sensitivity for metastatic detection by imaging occurs through:
   a. I-123 MIBG only
   b. Bone scan only
   c. Combination of I-123 MIBG and bone scan
   d. Combination of I-123 and In-111 Octreoscan

Case 124

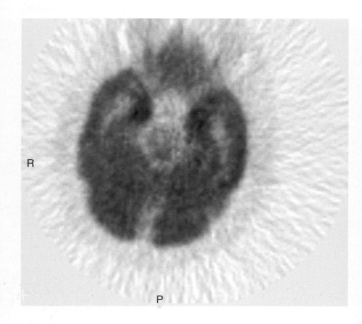

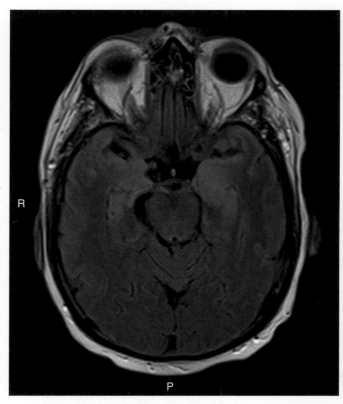

1. What is the salient finding on the F-18 FDG-PET brain study section shown?
   a. Abnormal increased activity in the medial temporal lobes
   b. Abnormal increased activity in the right medial temporal lobe
   c. Abnormal decreased activity in the left medial temporal lobe
   d. Abnormal decreased activity in the right medial temporal lobe
2. What is the most likely diagnosis in a patient with an acute change in mental status?
   a. Limbic encephalitis
   b. Metastases
   c. Mesial temporal sclerosis
   d. Ganglioglioma
3. What antibody is associated with autoimmune encephalitis in young women with a history of teratomas?
   a. Anti-NMDA (N methyl aspartic acid)
   b. Anti-VGKC (voltage-gated potassium channel)
   c. Anti-GAD (glutamic acid decarboxylase)
   d. Anti-GABA (gamma aminobutyric acid)
4. In a patient with these images and a clinical history of acute onset and fever what diagnosis should be strongly considered?
   a. Herpes simplex encephalitis
   b. Toxoplasmosis
   c. Neurocysticercosis
   d. Low-grade astrocytoma

Case 125

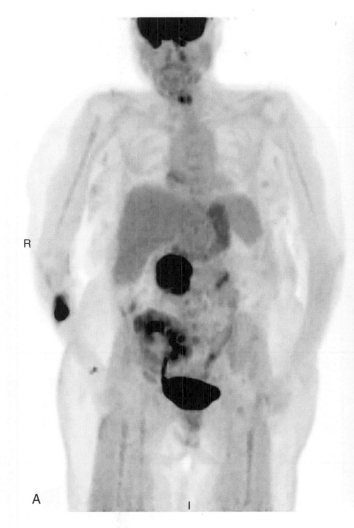

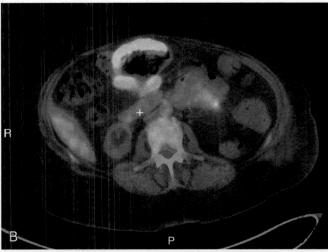

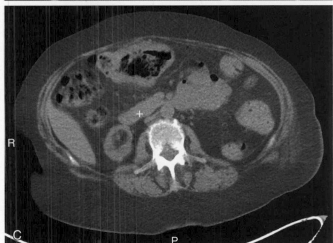

1. What are the salient findings?
   a. Right pelvic mass and midabdominal mass
   b. Physiologic activity in the right pelvis and mass in the midabdomen
   c. Physiologic activity in the right pelvis and midabdomen
   d. Right pelvic mass and physiologic activity in the midabdomen

2. What is the most likely diagnosis given the constellation of findings?
   a. Colon cancer
   b. Ptotic kidney
   c. Post-transplantation lymphoproliferative disease (PTLD)
   d. Renal cell cancer

3. Which body compartment is most likely to be involved?
   a. Neck
   b. Chest
   c. Abdomen
   d. Pelvis

4. PTLD occurrence is associated with which of the following?
   a. Epstein-Barr virus (EBV)
   b. Herpes simplex virus
   c. Norovirus
   d. Cytomegalovirus (CMV)

Case 126

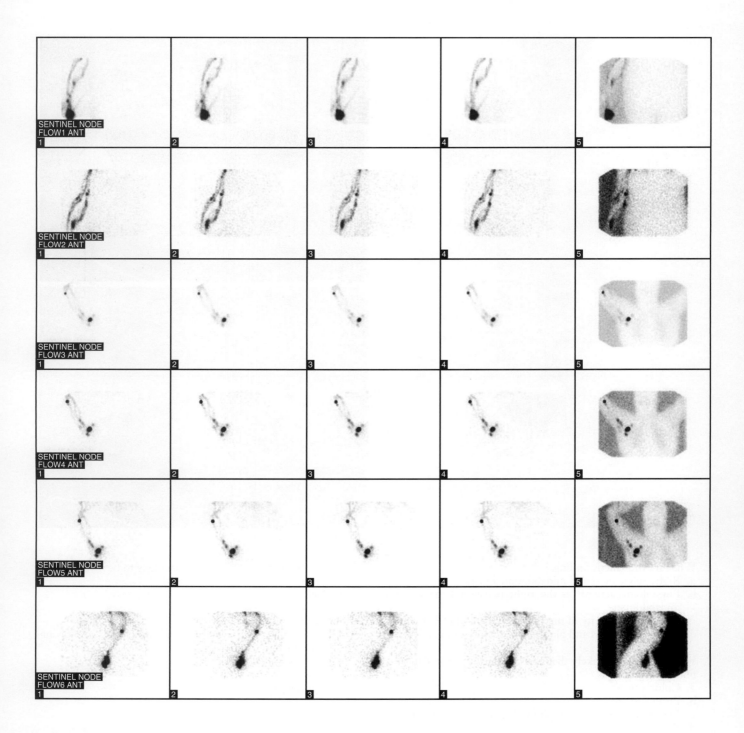

1. What kind of study is this?
   a. Lymphoscintigraphy
   b. Cystography
   c. Milk study
   d. Thyroid scan
2. What is the diagnosis?
   a. Lymphatic leak
   b. Neoplastic lesion in the antecubital fossa
   c. Epitrochlear lymph node
   d. Lymphatic obstruction
3. Why are these studies performed?
   a. To identify foci of disease
   b. To evaluate for lymphatic spread of disease
   c. To identify the sentinel node for surgical planning
   d. For post op evaluation of lymph node dissections
4. Which area does the epitrochlear lymph node station drain?
   a. Third through fifth fingers
   b. Thumb
   c. Axilla
   d. Subpectoral region

Case 127

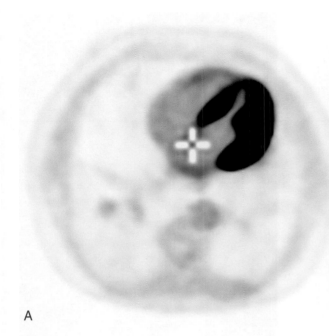

A

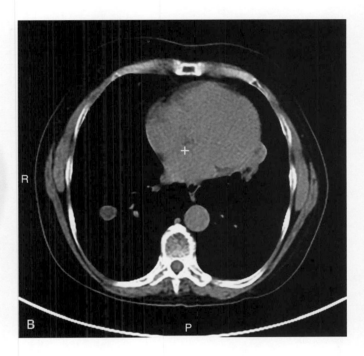

B

1. What is the salient finding?
   a. Benign-appearing lung nodule
   b. Spiculated FDG-avid lung nodule
   c. FDG-avid pulmonary infarct
   d. FDG-avid pleural effusion
2. What is the most likely diagnosis?
   a. Adenocarcinoma
   b. Pulmonary carcinoid
   c. Hamartoma
   d. Granuloma

3. Which entity is most likely to cause a false-negative result on FDG PET/CT?
   a. Colon carcinoma metastases
   b. Pulmonary carcinoid
   c. Small cell lung cancer
   d. Pulmonary infection/abscess
4. According to the 2017 Fleischner Society guidelines, for which nodule should a PET/CT considered?
   a. Single, solid, 4-mm nodule in a low-risk patient
   b. Single, solid, 6-mm nodule in a high-risk patient
   c. Multiple, solid, 6-mm nodules in a high-risk patient
   d. Single, solid, 9-mm nodule in a low-risk patient

Case 128

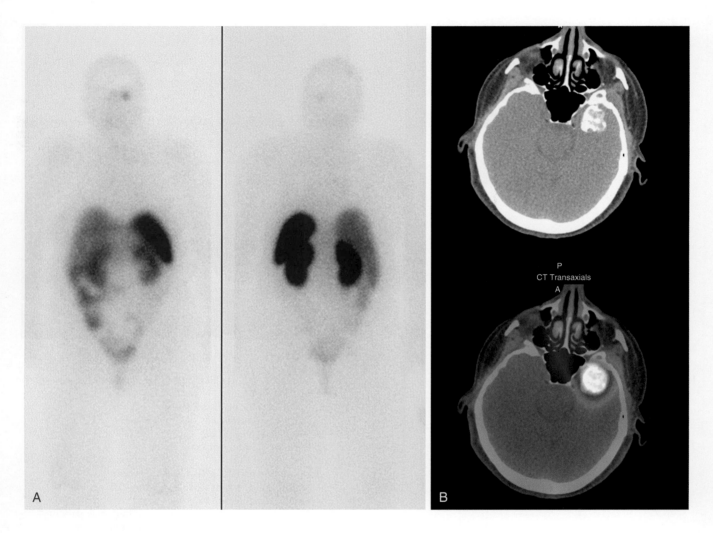

A

P
CT Transaxials
A

B

1. What is the radiopharmaceutical?
   a. In-111 WBC
   b. Ga-67 citrate
   c. In-111 Octreoscan
   d. Tc-99m MDP bone scan
2. What is the abnormality?
   a. Inadequate excretion of radiotracer from the kidneys
   b. Intestinal uptake
   c. Focal uptake in the cranium
   d. Focal lesion in the liver
3. What is the most likely diagnosis?
   a. Glioblastoma multiforme
   b. Meningioma
   c. Metastases
   d. Meningitis
4. What other tumors might be diagnosed by using this radio-pharmaceutical?
   a. Carcinoid of the lung
   b. Non–small cell lung cancer
   c. Renal cell carcinoma
   d. Colon cancer

Case 129

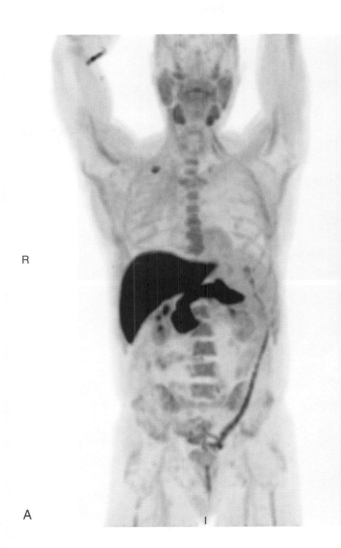

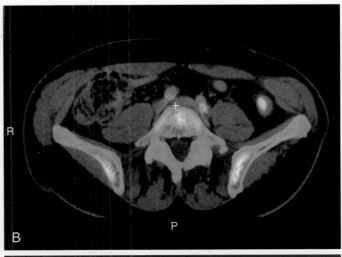

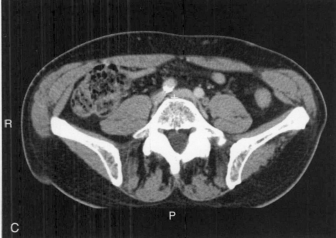

1. What is the radiopharmaceutical?
   a. F-18 FDG
   b. F-18 florbetapir
   c. F-18 NaF
   d. F-18 Fluciclovine
2. What is likely underlying diagnosis?
   a. Pancreatic cancer
   b. Multiple myeloma
   c. Prostate cancer
   d. Colon cancer

3. Why is F-18 FDG PET/CT of limited utility in the workup of prostate cancer?
   a. Low glucose utilization of the tumor
   b. Physiologic bowel uptake obscures tumor
   c. Adenocarcinomas tend not to be FDG avid
   d. Short half-life of F-18
4. What is the mechanism of action of this radiopharmaceutical?
   a. Amino acid transportation
   b. Glucose utilization
   c. Plaque deposition
   d. Chemadsorption

Case 130

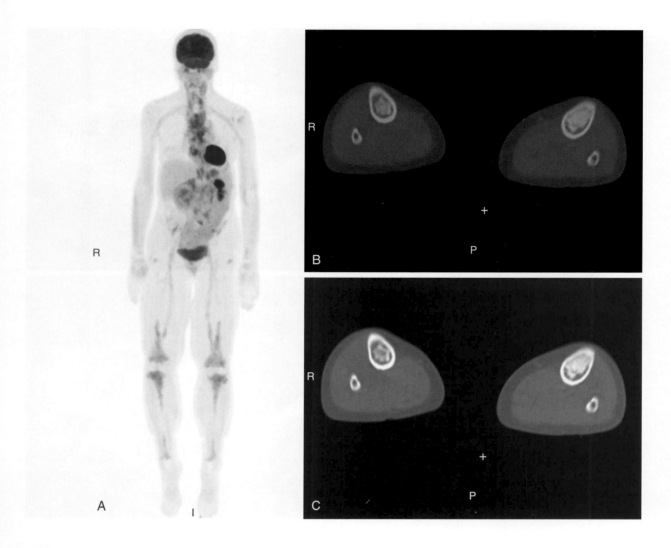

1. What is the salient finding?
   a. Sclerosis in the long bones of the lower extremities associated with increased FDG activity
   b. Sclerosis in the long bone of the lower extremities associated with decreased FDG activity
   c. Abnormal FDG activity in soft tissues
   d. No focal abnormality
2. What is the most likely diagnosis?
   a. Multiple endocrine neoplasia (MEN) I
   b. Erdheim-Chester disease
   c. Paget's disease
   d. Eosinophilic granulomatosis
3. What is the most common clinical symptom?
   a. Arrhythmia
   b. Seizure
   c. Bone pain
   d. Renal failure
4. All of the following are potential therapies EXCEPT:
   a. Steroids
   b. Antiestrogens
   c. Chemotherapy
   d. Radiation

Case 131

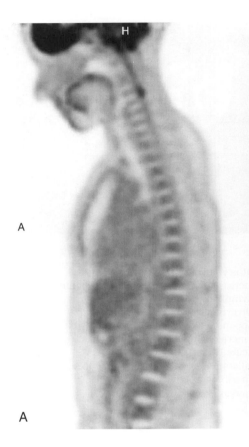

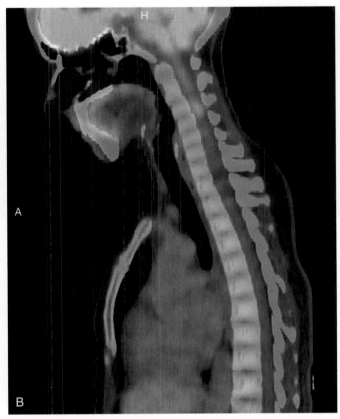

1. What is the salient finding in this patient who recently received a vaccination?
   a. Increased FDG uptake in the osseous structures
   b. Increased FDG uptake in the frontal lobes
   c. Absent FDG uptake in the myocardium
   d. Focal uptake in the cervical spinal cord
2. What is the expected appearance of the cervical spinal cord on a normal FDG PET/CT scan?
   a. No FDG uptake
   b. Uniform uptake that gradually fades caudally
   c. Focal uptake at C6/7
   d. Multifocal, patchy uptake extending to the lower thoracic cord

3. What is the next step in the imaging workup of this patient?
   a. CT scan of the cervical spine
   b. MRI of the cervical spine
   c. CT myelography
   d. Biopsy
4. In a patient with a history of recent immunization, what is the most likely diagnosis?
   a. Metastatic disease
   b. Glioblastoma multiforme
   c. Transverse myelitis
   d. Infarction

Case 132

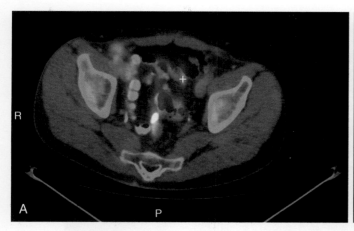
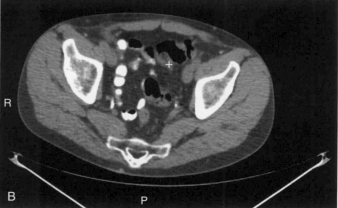

1. What is the salient finding?
   a. Focal FDG activity in the right inguinal canal associated with a soft tissue density
   b. Focal FDG activity in a ureter
   c. Physiologic muscle activity
   d. Physiologic bowel activity
2. What is the most likely etiology in a patient with a history of recent surgery?
   a. Inflammatory healing response to recent surgery
   b. Lymphadenopathy
   c. Physiologic bowel uptake
   d. Inflammatory changes related to the appendix
3. What is your interpretation?
   a. Increased FDG uptake in a hernia plug repair
   b. Lymphoma
   c. Diverticulitis
   d. Appendicitis
4. The increased uptake is most likely related to:
   a. Acute bacterial infection
   b. Inflammatory change related to foreign object
   c. Physiologic activity
   d. Increased glycolysis in tumor cells

Case 133

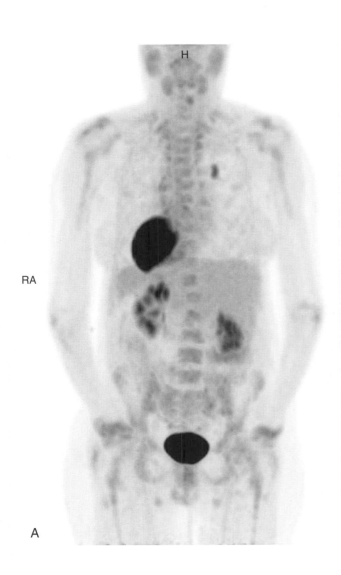

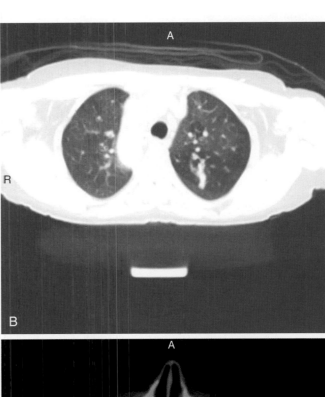

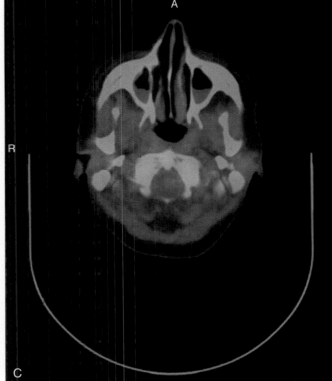

1. What is the most likely diagnosis?
   a. Kartagener's syndrome
   b. Osler-Weber-Rendu syndrome
   c. Mazabraud's syndrome
   d. Cowden's syndrome

2. What is the primary pathology that results in clinical symptoms?
   a. Ciliary dyskinesia
   b. Amyloid plaque deposition
   c. Vascular malformations
   d. Multiple hamartomas

3. What are the most common clinical symptoms?
   a. Heart failure
   b. Liver failure
   c. Chronic infection
   d. Intestinal obstruction caused by the presence of tumoral growths

4. What is the etiology for this finding?
   a. CMV exposure
   b. Autosomal dominant inheritance
   c. Autosomal recessive inheritance
   d. EBV exposure

Case 134

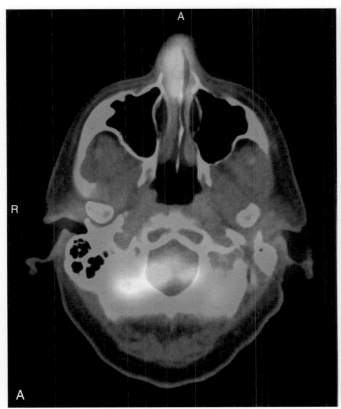

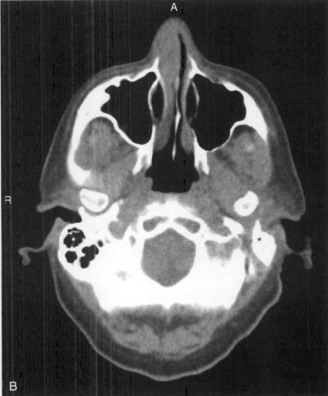

1. What is the most likely etiology for this abnormality?
   a. Sinonasal malignancy
   b. Acute infection
   c. Rhinorrhea
   d. Physiologic activity
2. What is the most common histopathology for sinonasal lymphoma?
   a. T-cell lymphoma
   b. Mucosa-associated lymphoid tissue (MALT) lymphoma
   c. Diffuse large cell B cell lymphoma
   d. Hodgkin's disease

3. What is the best imaging modality for assessing locoregional disease?
   a. Ultrasonography (US)
   b. CT
   c. MRI
   d. PET/CT
4. What is the likely treatment for this entity?
   a. Antibiotics
   b. Surgery
   c. Radiation only
   d. Combination of radiation and chemotherapy

Case 135

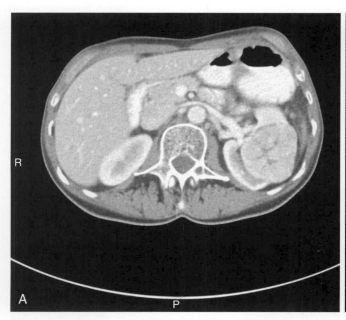
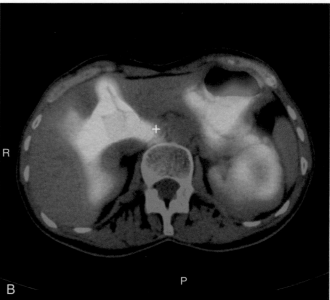

1. What is the finding on the contrast-enhanced CT scan?
   a. Left adrenal mass
   b. Left renal mass
   c. Retroperitoneal adenopathy
   d. Abnormal perfusion to the left kidney relative to the right kidney
2. Why was the renal Tc-99m sestamibi study performed?
   a. To characterize the abnormality as benign/indolent versus malignant
   b. To evaluate for additional site of disease
   c. To assess differential renal function
   d. To assess for renal obstruction
3. What is the most likely diagnosis?
   a. Oncocytoma
   b. Renal cell carcinoma
   c. Hematoma
   d. Paraganglioma
4. What is the likely explanation for the radiotracer uptake?
   a. Increased perfusion to the lesion
   b. Increased density of mitochondria within the lesion
   c. Trapping within in the cell as a result of phosphorylation
   d. Preferential renal excretion

Case 136

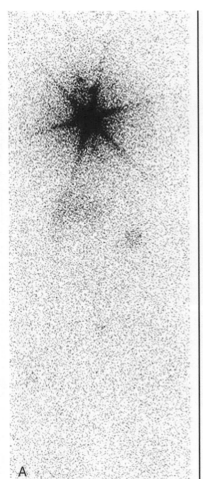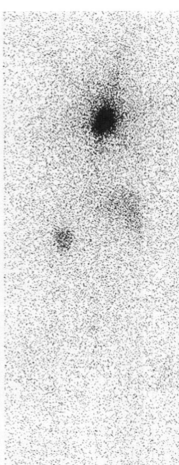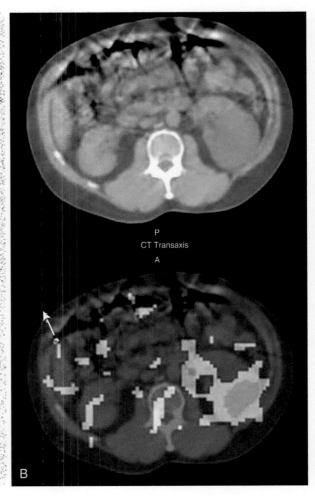

1. What is the radiotracer?
   a. I-131
   b. I-123 MIBG
   c. In-111 Octreoscan
   d. I-123

2. What is the most salient unexpected abnormality?
   a. Increased uptake in the neck
   b. Focal uptake in the lungs suggestive of metastases
   c. Bowel activity
   d. Focal activity in the left midabdomen

3. What is the reason for this finding in this patient?
   a. Renal excretion of radiotracer
   b. Accumulation of radiotracer in the left kidney
   c. Renal metastases
   d. Bowel activity

4. What is the most likely time point for this scan in a patient being treated for papillary thyroid cancer?
   a. Pre–I-131 therapy
   b. 1 day after I-131 therapy
   c. A week after I-131 therapy
   d. 1 year follow-up

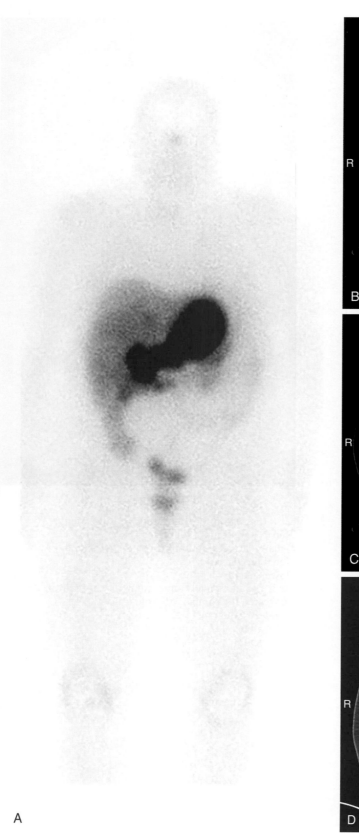

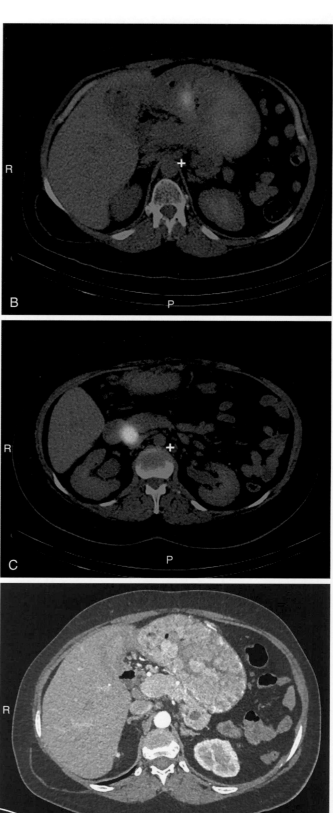

1. What is the radiopharmaceutical?
    a. F-18 FDG
    b. Tc-99m pertechnetate
    c. In-111 Octreoscan
    d. Tc-99m mebrofenin
2. What is the salient finding?
    a. Physiologic activity in the stomach
    b. Abnormal radiotracer uptake in the stomach
    c. Focal liver lesion
    d. Splenic infarct
3. In a patient with history of MEN1, what is the likely diagnosis?
    a. Gastric carcinoid
    b. Gastritis
    c. Gastric lymphoma
    d. Physiologic uptake
4. Type I gastric carcinoid is most commonly associated with:
    a. Chronic atrophic gastritis
    b. Gastric ulcers
    c. Pheochromocytomas
    d. MEN 1

Case 138

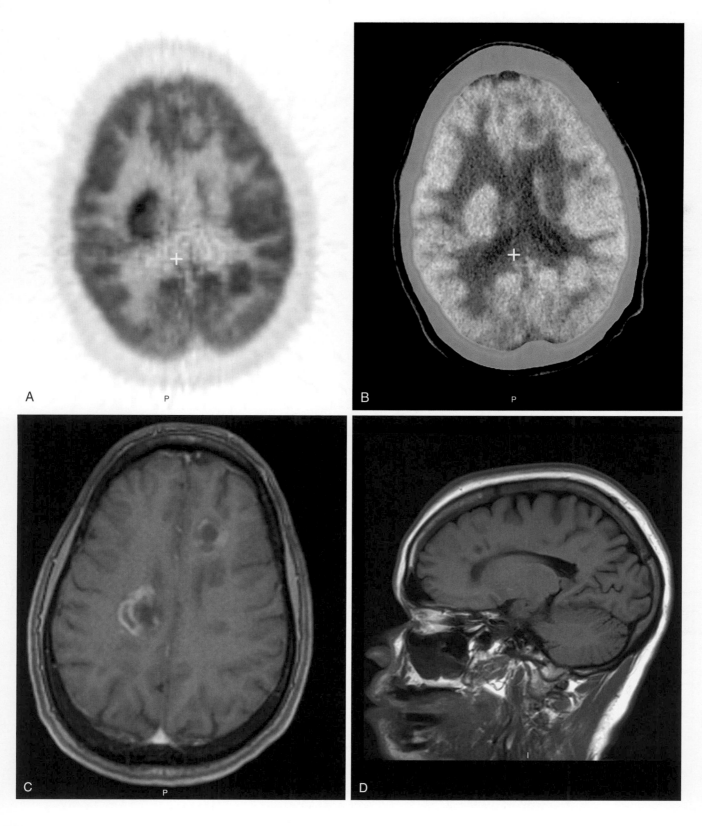

1. What are the salient findings?
   a. FDG-avid white matter lesions
   b. Physiologic activity
   c. FDG-avid skull lesions
   d. Focal cortical metabolically active lesions
2. Given the MRI findings above, what do you think is the likely diagnosis?
   a. Tumefactive multiple sclerosis (MS)
   b. Metastases
   c. Seizures
   d. Oligodendroglioma
3. What is the pathologic hallmark for MS?
   a. Necrosis
   b. Demyelination
   c. Amyloid plaque presence
   d. Neurofibrillary tangles
4. What is likely the etiology for increased FDG uptake?
   a. Physiologic activity
   b. Chronic plaque formation
   c. Treatment response
   d. Active inflammation

Case 139

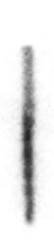

A

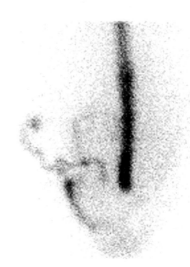

B

Image A is from the patient's prior study. Image B is from the patient's present study.

1. In a patient who has had surgery for pseudotumor cerebri, what kind of study is this?
   a. Lumboperitoneal (LP) shunt patency evaluation
   b. Ventriculoperitoneal (VP) shunt patency evaluation
   c. Ventriculopleural shunt patency evaluation
   d. Radionuclide cisternography
2. What is the likely radiotracer?
   a. Tc-99m DTPA
   b. Tc-99m HMPAO
   c. Tc-99m MAG3
   d. Tc-99m pertechnetate

3. What is the diagnosis for Image A?
   a. CSF leak
   b. Obstructed LP shunt catheter
   c. Patent LP shunt catheter
   d. Obstructed VP shunt catheter
4. What imaging finding would be indicative of LP shunt patency?
   a. Radiotracer activity confined within the spinal column
   b. No radiotracer activity within the spinal column
   c. Free flow of radiotracer within the peritoneum
   d. Reflux of radiotracer into the ventricular system

Case 140

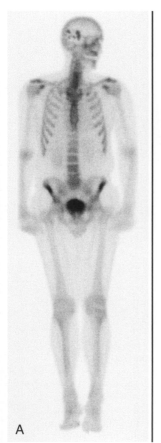
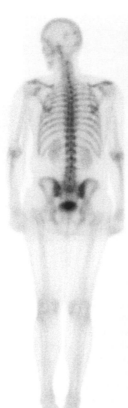
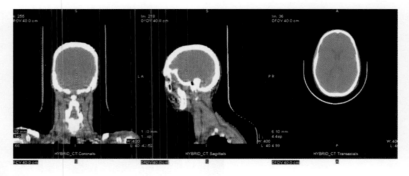
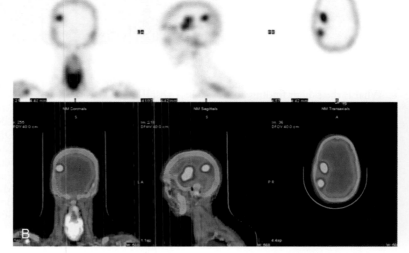

1. What is the salient finding on the bone scan single photon-emission computed tomography/CT (SPECT/CT)?
   a. Skull metastases
   b. Focal uptake in the cerebrum
   c. Physiologic radiotracer activity
   d. Intraventricular lesion
2. What is the next step in evaluating this patient?
   a. MRI of the brain
   b. CT of the pelvis
   c. Renal US
   d. No follow-up needed—contamination

3. What is the likely diagnosis?
   a. Infarct
   b. Tumor
   c. Aneurysm
   d. Physiologic uptake
4. Which entity may cause Tc-99m MDP uptake in the brain?
   a. Infarct
   b. Tumor
   c. Encephalitis
   d. All of the above

Case 141

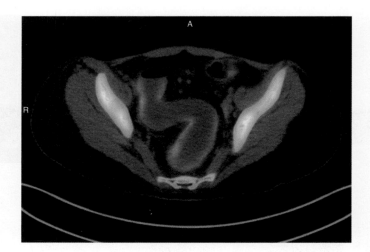

1. What is the salient finding on this F-18 FDG PET/CT scan?
   a. Featureless colon
   b. Perirectal lymphadenopathy
   c. Rectosigmoid malignancy
   d. Diverticulitis
2. What is the name of this radiographic sign?
   a. Sandwich sign
   b. Scimitar sign
   c. Lead pipe sign
   d. String sign
3. What is the likely diagnosis?
   a. Crohn's disease
   b. Ulcerative colitis
   c. Diverticulosis
   d. Colonic polyposis
4. Patients with this disease are at increased risk for:
   a. Perforation
   b. Malignancy
   c. Bowel obstruction
   d. Splenic infarct

Case 142

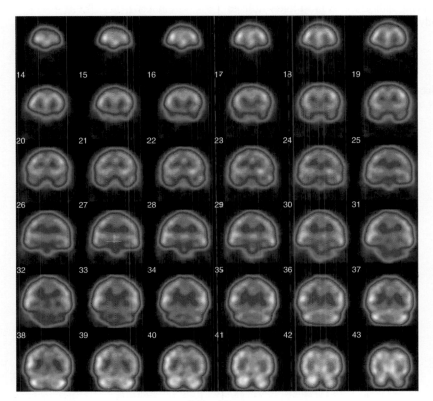

(A) Ictal Scan

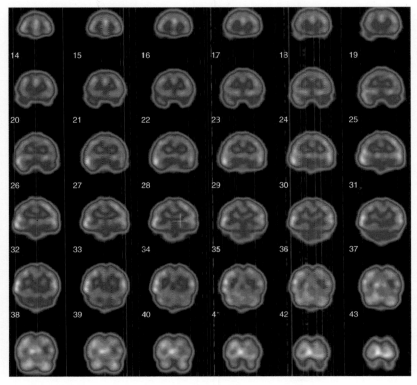

(B) Interictal Scan

1. Where is the seizure focus?
   a. Left frontal lobe
   b. Right frontal lobe
   c. Right temporal lobe
   d. Left temporal lobe
2. Which one of the following radiotracer is most likely utilized for a SPECT ictal study?
   a. Tc-99m DTPA
   b. Tc-99 HMPAO
   c. F-18 FDG
   d. F-18 amyloid
3. When performing an ictal SPECT study, the radiotracer should be injected within how many minutes of onset of seizure?
   a. 1 minute
   b. 5 minutes
   c. 10 minutes
   d. 15 minutes
4. The characteristic finding for a seizure focus on an ictal/interictal SPECT study is:
   a. Mismatch (decreased uptake on interictal/increased uptake on ictal)
   b. Mismatch (increased uptake on interictal/decreased uptake on ictal)
   c. Matched cold defects
   d. Matched hot defects

Case 143

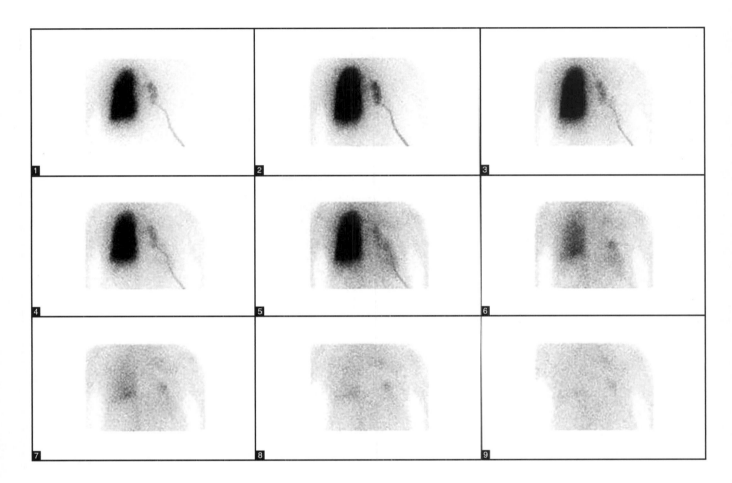

The patient recently underwent pneumonectomy, developed a post operative effusion, for which a drainage catheter was placed. A Xenon-133 ventilation study was performed.

1. The most likely diagnosis is:
   a. Bronchopleural fistula
   b. Pulmonary embolism
   c. Lung cancer
   d. Swyer-James syndrome
2. What is the physical half-life of Xe-133?
   a. 6 hours
   b. 13 hours
   c. 2.8 days
   d. 5.3 days

3. The photopeak for Xe-133 is:
   a. 81 keV
   b. 140 keV
   c. 159 keV
   d. 173 keV
4. The most common cause for this diagnosis is:
   a. Chemotherapy
   b. Infection
   c. Pneumothorax
   d. Lung resection

Case 144

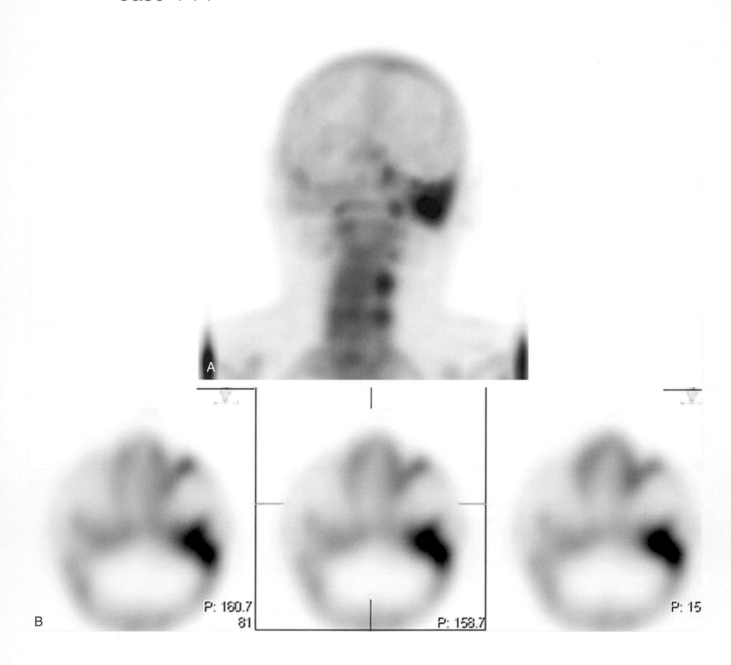

1. What is the salient finding on this bone scan?
   a. Focal uptake in the region of the left mastoid air cell/left external ear
   b. Focal uptake in the cervical spine
   c. Absence of brain activity
   d. Lack of radiotracer uptake in the right mastoid air cells/right external ear
2. What is the most likely diagnosis in a patient with ear pain and underlying diabetes mellitus?
   a. Metastases
   b. Malignant external otitis
   c. Paraganglioma
   d. Nasopharyngeal cancer
3. What is the most likely organism?
   a. *Pseudomonas*
   b. *Staphylococcus aureus*
   c. *Streptococcus*
   d. *Staphylococcus epidermis*
4. What other radiotracer may be used for the evaluation of suspected mastoiditis/malignant external otitis?
   a. Ga-68 DOTA-TATE
   b. Ga-67 citrate
   c. I-123 MIBG
   d. In-111 Octreoscan

Case 145

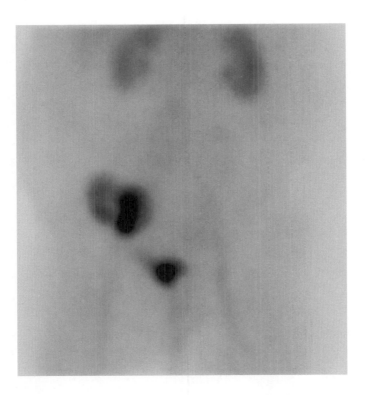

1. What is the most likely diagnosis?
   a. Renal infarct
   b. Vasomotor nephropathy
   c. Renal en bloc transplantation
   d. Decreased perfusion to the superior portion of a transplanted kidney
2. What is the most likely radiopharmaceutical utilized?
   a. Tc-99m MAG3
   b. Tc-99m DSMA
   c. Tc-99m pertechnetate
   d. Tc-99m mebrofenin
3. What is the imaging characteristic differentiating acute renal rejection from vasomotor nephropathy?
   a. Acute renal rejection has preserved flow, whereas flow is decreased in the setting of vasomotor nephropathy.
   b. Vasomotor nephropathy has preserved flow, whereas acute rejection demonstrates decreased flow.
   c. Acute rejection is characterized by no radiotracer excretion, whereas vasomotor nephropathy has normal excretion of radiotracer.
   d. The characteristics cannot be differentiated.
4. When would you expect to see bladder activity in a normally functioning single renal transplant?
   a. Immediately
   b. 4–8 minutes
   c. 10–20 minutes
   d. Greater than 20 minutes

Case 146

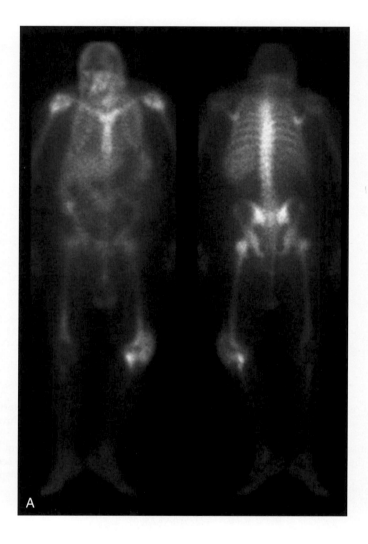

A

1. What is the half-life of Ga-67?
   a. 6 hours
   b. 13 hours
   c. 67 hours
   d. 78 hours
2. What are the primary photopeaks for Ga-67?
   a. 93 keV, 184 keV, 296 keV, 388 keV
   b. 93 keV, 140 keV, 247 keV, 301 keV
   c. 33 keV, 140 keV, 247 keV, 388 keV
   d. 33 keV, 184 keV, 296 keV, 301 keV

3. What is the ideal time point for imaging when assessing for infection?
   a. 3 hours
   b. 12 hours
   c. 24 hours
   d. 72 hours
4. To what protein does Ga-67 bind to in the blood pool?
   a. Albumin
   b. Transferrin
   c. Hemoglobin
   d. Fibrinogen

Case 147

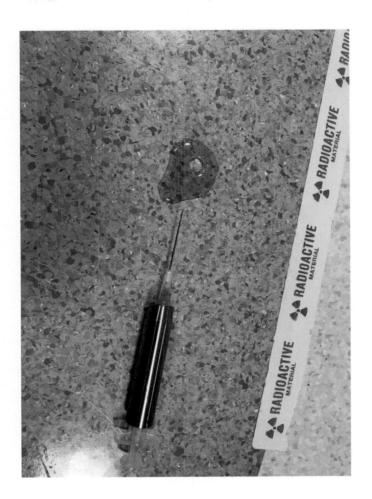

1. What is the threshold for a major spill of Tc-99m?
   a. 1 mCi
   b. 10 mCi
   c. 100 mCi
   d. 1000 mCi
2. What is the threshold for a major spill of I-131?
   a. 1 mCi
   b. 10 mCi
   c. 100 mCi
   d. 1000 mCi

3. What is the threshold for a major spill of I-123?
   a. 1 mCi
   b. 10 mCi
   c. 100 mCi
   d. 1000 mCi
4. All of the following guidelines should be followed if 5 mCi of Ga-67 is spilled EXCEPT:
   a. Report to radiation safety officer (RSO)
   b. Notify Nuclear Regulatory Commission (NRC)
   c. Contain with absorbent paper
   d. Wear gloves and gowns when cleaning up the area

Case 148

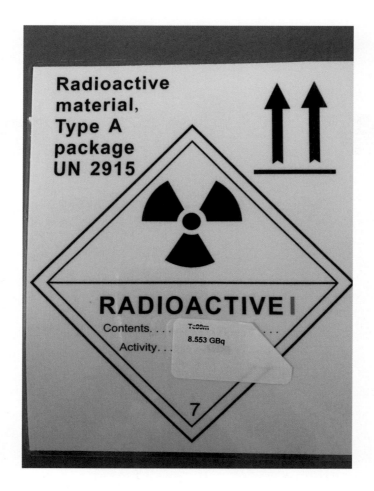

1. Packages containing radionuclides must be monitored and surveyed:
   a. Immediately upon receipt
   b. Within 3 hours of receipt or 3 hours of opening of the next business day
   c. Within 8 hours of receipt or 8 hours of opening of the next business day
   d. Do not need to be surveyed
2. External measurements of a package must be performed:
   a. On the surface
   b. At 1 cm distance
   c. At 1 m distance
   d. A and C

3. What does the "8.553 GBq" signify in the image above?
   a. The radionuclide dose
   b. The radionuclide dose expected at the time of injection
   c. The number of millirems per hour measured at 1 m from the package
   d. The number of millirems per hour measured at the surface
4. What does "Radioactive I" signify?
   a. No special handling is required. The surface dose may not exceed 0.5 mrem/hr.
   b. Special handling is required. The surface dose may not exceed 50 mrem/hr.
   c. Special handling is required. The surface dose may not exceed 100 mrem/hr.
   d. Special handling is required. The surface dose may not exceed 200 mrem/hr.

Case 149

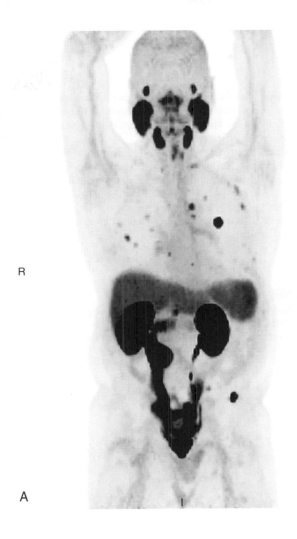

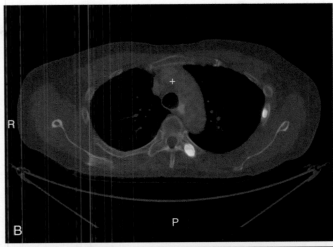

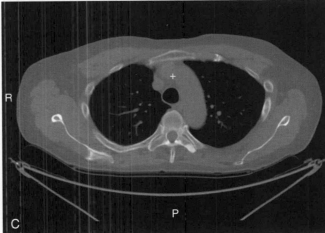

1. In this patient with a history of prostate cancer, what is the radiopharmaceutical used for this scan?
   a. F-18 FDG
   b. F-18 NaF
   c. F-18 PSMA
   d. Ga-68 DOTA-TATE
2. What is the physiologic target for this radiopharmaceutical?
   a. Somatostatin receptors
   b. Prostate specific membrane antigen
   c. Mitochondria
   d. CD20

3. All of the following radiopharmaceuticals have been used in the evaluation of patients with prostate cancer EXCEPT:
   a. F-18 FACBC
   b. Carbon-11 (C-11) choline
   c. Ga-68 PSMA
   d. C-11 PIB
4. Salivary gland uptake is:
   a. Physiologic
   b. Caused by fibrosis
   c. Caused by metastases
   d. Caused by iodine uptake

Case 1

THYROID—GRAVES' DISEASE

1. a
2. b
3. d
4. d

Discussion

Graves' disease is an autoimmune disease caused by a thyrotropin receptor antibody that stimulates thyroid follicular cells, resulting in excess production of thyroid hormone. It may manifest as anxiety, weight loss, exophthalmos, sweating, fatigue, fine tremor, and tachycardia.

The clinical diagnosis is confirmed with the finding of suppressed serum thyroid-stimulating hormone (TSH). The classic scintigraphic findings include diffuse increased radioactive iodine uptake in an enlarged thyroid gland with reduced background activity (as in this case). The pyramidal lobe is often visualized on a thyroid scan in a patient with Graves' disease. Subacute thyroiditis has low radioactive iodine uptake during the hyperthyroid phase because of suppressed TSH and normal pituitary feedback. Hot nodules are not seen on this study.

Symptoms may be controlled with beta blockers or antithyroid drugs (propylthiouracil or methimazole). Four- and 24-hour uptakes tend to be moderately to markedly elevated, 50% to 80%, respectively.

Definitive treatment includes I-131 therapy. Two different approaches may be utilized when selecting a dose. One school of thought gives a standard dose to all comers, usually between 10 to 15 mCi, whereas others calculate a dose based on gland size and percent uptake. If the patient has significant exophthalmos, pretreatment with steroid should be considered to prevent exacerbation of orbitopathy.

Surgery is not a standard treatment modality for Graves' disease.

REFERENCES

Lind P. Strategies of radioiodine therapy for Graves' disease. *Eur J Nuc Med.* 2002;29(suppl 2):453–457.

Ross DS, Burch HB, Cooper DS, et al. 2016 American Thyroid Association guidelines for diagnosis and management of hyperthyroidism and other causes of thyrotoxicosis. *Thyroid.* 2016;26(10):1343–1421.

Case 2

BONE SCAN—PROSTATE CANCER

1. d
2. a
3. b
4. c

Discussion

Bone scintigraphy is a sensitive method for the detection of osseous metastases. The bone scan is most sensitive when the serum prostate-specific antigen (PSA) level is greater than 20 ng/mL. However, PSA levels may not be elevated in patients with prostate cancer who have undergone hormone therapy. Approximately 80% of osseous metastatic lesions occur in the pelvic and axial skeleton. In advanced disease, lesions are seen in the skull and appendicular skeleton.

The primary finding on this bone scan (image A) is metastatic prostate cancer. The follow-up bone scan can also be described as a superscan because there is no renal or soft tissue uptake. This is due to extensive osseous metastases. Not all cases of a superscan resulting from metastases are so clear-cut. If the tumor has spread more diffusely through the entire skeleton, it may look similar to a superscan caused by underlying metabolic disease (e.g., renal disease or hyperparathyroidism). The clue to the diagnosis of metastases is that there is usually some focality or asymmetry to the pattern of uptake. Fluorine-18 (F-18) fluciclovine has been approved by the U.S. Food and Drug Administration (FDA) for the diagnosis of recurrent prostate cancer in patients with elevated PSA after prior therapy. It is an analogue of an amino acid. Amino acid transport is upregulated in prostate carcinoma. Indium-111 (In-111) capromab pendetide (ProstaScint) is a radiolabeled monoclonal antibody to prostate-specific membrane antigen that is imaged with a gamma camera, not positron emission–computed tomography (PET/CT) (Figures 2AB)

REFERENCES

Love C, Din AS, Tomas MB, Kalapparambath TP, Palestro CJ. Radionuclide bone imaging: an illustrative review. *Radiographics*. 2003;23(2):341–358.

Schuster DM, Nanni C, Fanti S. PET tracers beyond FDG in prostate cancer. *Semin Nucl Med*. 2016;46(6):507–521.

Walkitt KL, Khan SR, Dubash S, et al. Clinical PET imaging in prostate cancer. *Radiographics*. 2017;37(5):1512–1536.

Case 3

BRAIN DEATH

1. b
2. c
3. b
4. b

Discussion

Lack of blood flow to the brain is diagnostic of brain death. Only a minority of patients with suspected brain death are referred for this study (e.g., those with uncertain confirmatory test results, such as with electroencephalography [EEG], which may not be interpretable in the setting of barbiturate therapy or hypothermia). Although flow images by themselves (e.g., with technetium-99m (Tc-99m) diethylenetriaminepentaacetic acid [DTPA]) can often make the diagnosis, the results are susceptible to potential technical errors (e.g., starting the acquisition late or its malfunction during the flow phase). Tc-99m hexamethylpropylene amine oxime (HMPAO) or Tc-99m ethyl cysteinate dimer (ECD) are the preferred radiopharmaceutical because delayed static images can be obtained. These agents fix in the brain, and postflow images are diagnostic, usually acquired at 15 to 20 minutes, but timing is not critical. Normal blood flow findings include visualization in the intracranial arterial vasculature, including the middle cerebral artery (MCA) and the anterior cerebral artery (ACA), followed by cortical visualization and venous drainage in the sagittal and transverse sinuses. Lack of cerebral blood flow may result in the "hot nose sign" as blood flow is shunted from the internal carotid circulation to the external circulation (see Figure C). If no cerebral blood flow is present, there will be no uptake of radiotracer within the cerebrum or cerebellum. Brain perfusion scintigraphy is not affected by hypothermia or drugs.

REFERENCE

Laurin NR, Driedger AA, Hurwitz GA, et al. Cerebral perfusion imaging with technetium-99m HM-PAO in brain death and severe central nervous system injury. *Journal of Nuclear Medicine: Official Publication of the Society of Nuclear Medicine*. 1989;30(10):1627–1635.

Case 4

CARDIAC MUGA STUDY—ABNORMAL

1. c
2. b
3. b
4. a

Discussion

Radionuclide ventriculography, commonly called a *MUGA* scan (multigated acquisition), is performed to assess ventricular contraction and to calculate the left ventricular ejection fraction (LVEF). The study is performed by reinjecting the patient's own Tc-99m–labeled red blood cells (RBCs). This case shows the quantification of LVEF. A region of interest (ROI) is drawn in the left anterior oblique (LAO) projection because this renders a clear separation of the left ventricle from the right ventricle and adjacent cardiac structures and vessels. A background ROI is also drawn. LVEF is defined as the fraction of end-diastolic volume ejected from the left ventricle, or LVEF = end-diastolic counts – end-systolic counts/end-diastolic counts, corrected for background. The calculation is for the summed counts over many cardiac cycles. The MUGA study is gated to the electrocardiography (ECG) rhythm strip. Sixteen frames (bins) of data are acquired during each R-to-R interval and then summed over about 300 cycles. Calculation of an accurate LVEF is dependent on a normal rhythm or at least only a mild arrhythmia. LVEF calculations may be erroneous in patients with irregular heartbeats, because data will be misplaced in the sequential 16 frames (bins). The time activity curve (ventricular volume curve) in the right lower corner should be reviewed. It should start and end at the same point. If not, there is likely a gating problem. The color images of the heart are functional images, which are beyond the scope of this discussion. The phase histogram in the center of the page demonstrates two peaks, suggesting an arrhythmia. There should be only a single peak.

This study demonstrates a decreased LVEF (30%) in a patient receiving doxorubicin (Adriamycin) therapy. Anthracycline drugs, such as doxorubicin, are commonly used to treat malignancies, such as lymphoma or breast cancer. The drug is known to cause left ventricular function depression related to cumulative dose effect. Trastuzumab (Herceptin) may also cause cardiac toxicity. There are specific criteria related the LVEF with regard to reducing the drug or stopping it if the LVEF is reduced.

REFERENCES

Fatima N, Zaman M, Hashmi A, Kamal S, Hameed A. Assessing adriamycin-induced early cardiotoxicity by estimating left ventricular ejection fraction using technetium-99m multiple-gated acquisition scan and echocardiography. *Nucl Med Commun*. 2011;32(5):381–385.

Slamon DJ, Leyland-Jones B, Shak S, et al. Concurrent administration of anti-HER2 monoclonal antibody and first-line chemotherapy for HER2-overexpressing metastatic breast cancer. A phase III, multinational, randomized controlled trial. *N Engl J Med*. 2001;344(11):783–792.

Nicol A, Avison M, Harbinson M, et al. Procedure guideline for planar radionuclide cardiac ventriculogram for the assessment of left ventricular systolic function. *Nucl Med Commun*. 2000;30(3):245–252.

Case 5

HIDA—BILIARY LEAK

1. d
2. a
3. a
4. c

Discussion

This case demonstrates the presence of a bile leak after cholecystectomy. There is radiotracer pooling in the right paracolic gutter as well as along the inferior margin of the right hepatic lobe. There are several possible etiologies for the occurrence of a bile leak, including liver transplantation, partial hepatectomy, an inflammatory condition, percutaneous interventions, trauma, and cholecystectomy.

Several studies have reported that the incidence of bile leak after laparoscopic cholecystectomy ranges from 1.1% to 11.3%. This is a serious complication that can result in peritonitis, abscess, and fistula formations. The most common clinical symptom reported is abdominal pain. The most common cause for a leak after cholecystectomy is breakdown of or incomplete ligation of the cystic duct. Postoperative fluid collections are often seen on computed tomography (CT). Hepatobiliary scanning can confirm whether these are biliary in origin. A slow leak may resolve on its own with supportive care, whereas a rapid leak will often require a second surgery.

Scintigraphy is a very sensitive, noninvasive method to clearly identify leaks and characterize their rate of leakage. The most common site for a biliary collection is the gallbladder fossa. The classic pattern of bile leak can be described as originating from the gallbladder fossa extending to the right paracolic gutter or over the dome of the liver. Bilomas may initially appear photopenic and, over time, demonstrate increase in radiotracer accumulation. Delayed imaging up to 24 hours may be beneficial for detecting slow leaks or collection obscured by tracer within the bowel. In patients with a complex surgical history, a single-photon emission computed tomography SPECT/CT may add value by clearly localizing radiotracer uptake to collections seen on CT.

REFERENCES

Barkun AN, Rezieg M, Mehta SN, et al. Postcholecystectomy biliary leaks in the laparoscopic era: risk factors, presentation, and management. McGill Gallstone Treatment Group. *Gastrointest Endosc*. 1997;45(3):277–282.

Hasl DM, Ruiz OR, Baumert J, et al. A prospective study of bile leaks after laparoscopic cholecystectomy. *Surg Endosc*. 2001;15(11):1299–1300.

Mujoomdar M, Russell E, Dionne F, et al. Optimizing health system use of medical isotopes and other imaging modalities [Internet]. *Ottawa (ON): Canadian Agency for Drugs and Technologies in Health*. 2012. APPENDIX 2.2, Detection of Bile Leak.

Case 6

GASTRIC EMPTYING—SOLID DELAYED

1. b
2. d
3. a
4. d

Discussion

The radionuclide gastric emptying study is considered the gold standard for the evaluation of gastric dysmotility. The 2008 Consensus Recommendations for Radionuclide Gastric Emptying Scintigraphy was published in an effort to standardize the test results across medical centers. The guidelines recommend a standard meal, comprised of 4 oz egg white substitute labeled with Tc-99m, two slices of toast, strawberry jam (30g), water (120 mL), and a simplified methodology of acquiring 1-minute images immediately after ingestion and at 1, 2, and 4 hours. The 4-hour imaging protocol was found to identify 30% more patients with gastroparesis compared with a 2-hour protocol. Normal values are based on a large published normal database: greater than 10% emptying at 1 hour, greater than 40% emptying at 2 hours, and greater than 90% emptying at 4 hours. These values are only truly applicable if the patient has eaten the entire meal. Smaller-volume meals are emptied faster. For quantification, ROIs are drawn around the acquired anterior and posterior images at each time point. The results must be corrected for decay and attenuation. The geometric mean (square root of the product of the anterior and posterior counts) method is considered the gold standard for correction method.

REFERENCES

Donohoe KJ, Maurer AH, Ziessman HA, et al. Procedure guideline for adult solid-meal gastric-emptying study 3.0. *J Nucl Med Technol.* 2009;37(3):196–200.

Ziessman HA, Goetze S, Bonta D, Ravich W. Experience with a new standardized 4-hr gastric emptying protocol. *J Nucl Med.* 2007;48(4):568–572.

Case 7

BONE SCAN—OSTEOMYELITIS

1. b
2. c
3. a
4. a

Discussion

Bone scintigraphy not only detects areas of osseous metastases but is also valuable for assessing the presence of benign bone diseases such as infections, fractures, and benign tumors. Tc-99 methyl diphosphonate (MDP) can be prepared by using a simple kit. Incomplete labeling may occur if air is introduced into the vial. The radiopharmaceutical should be used within 2 to 3 hours of preparation to avoid significant buildup of free pertechnetate from breakdown of the radiolabel.

Although the degree of bone uptake is related to blood flow, the most important factor is the amount of osteogenic activity. Osteogenic activity is higher in areas of bone repair and/or formation.

Osteomyelitis is often the result of overlying soft tissue infection or hematogenous seeding. The most common organism found in areas of osseous infection is *Staphylococcus aureus*.

The standard protocol for the evaluation of osteomyelitis is a three-phase bone scan, consisting of a flow phase (first 60 seconds after injection); early arterial flow seen in the first few seconds is characteristic, followed by a static blood pool image immediately after flow, and then a delayed image at 3 to 4 hours after injection to allow time for background clearance. In a patient with diabetes or severe edema, an additional fourth-phase image at 24 hours may be indicated for further reduction in soft tissue background activity and improved bone visualization.

Osteomyelitis is typically positive on all three phases. This is suggestive of, but not specific for, osteomyelitis and should be correlated with dedicated plain films to exclude the presence of fracture, Charcot joint, tumor, and so on that may also be three-phase positive.

Improved specificity can be obtained by performing a subsequent In-111 or Tc-99m leukocyte scan. False-negative results are infrequent but have been reported in infants and also in adults with vertebral infection. Falsely negative regions of infection may be seen as normal, reduced uptake, or photopenia (cold), which may be secondary to increased pressure in the marrow spaces or thrombosis of vessels.

REFERENCES

Annen MJ, Johnston MJ, Gormley JP, Silverman E. Acute hematogenous osteomyelitis presenting as a cold rib in a child. *World J Nucl Med*. 2017;16(2):160–162.

Palestro CJ. Radionuclide imaging of musculoskeletal infection. *J Nucl Med*. 2016;57(9):1406–1412.

Case 8

F-18 FDG PET—HOT THYROID NODULE

1. a
2. d
3. a
4. d

Discussion

Thyroid nodules are frequently identified on F-18 fluorodeoxy-glucose (FDG) PET/CT scans obtained for indications other than evaluation of the thyroid gland. Some of these nodules are FDG avid. The cancer risk of a focal FDG avid thyroid nodule is approximately 30%. A prudent follow-up to incidental detection of an FDG-avid thyroid nodule would be dedicated ultrasonography (US) of the thyroid gland and consideration of biopsy if sonographic characteristics are suspicious for malignancy.

REFERENCES

Bae JS, et al. Incidental thyroid lesions detected by FDG-PET/CT: prevalence and risk of thyroid cancer. *World J Surg Oncol.* 2009;7(1):63.

Case 9

BONE SCAN—INSUFFICIENCY FRACTURES

1. c
2. b
3. c
4. a

Discussion

This patient has the classic findings of sacral insufficiency fractures on a bone scan. On bone scans, sacral insufficiency fractures characteristically have an H-shaped appearance because of intense vertical uptake in the region of the sacroiliac joints and horizontal uptake in the mid-sacrum. Thus, this pattern of uptake is often referred to as the "H sign," or *Honda sign*.

Patients with sacral insufficiency fractures often are elderly individuals, with vague complaints that may delay detection. These often occur in the absence of known trauma or with minimal trauma. However, metastatic disease must be excluded with dedicated anatomic imaging, particularly in patients with a history of cancer. The most sensitive methods for radiologic detection are bone scintigraphy and magnetic resonance imaging (MRI). Recommended treatment options most commonly include conservative therapy (bed rest or moderation of activity) with pain analgesics. Minimally invasive techniques, such as sacroplasty, are being explored. Open surgery or chemotherapy is not indicated.

In this patient, multiple adjacent right anterior ribs also have uptake, suggesting fractures and underlying osteoporosis. There are multiple causes for osteoporosis, including hyperparathyroidism, Cushing's syndrome, therapy with corticosteroids, prior radiation therapy, treatment for prostate cancer to reduce testosterone, hyperthyroidism, and postmenopausal osteoporosis (the most common one).

Because of decreased bone mineral density, insufficiency fractures may be difficult to identify on plain-film radiographs. However, increased radiotracer activity is readily seen on bone scans because of increased osteoblastic activity and bone turnover. Common sites for osteoporosis-related fractures include the vertebral column, proximal femurs, ribs, and pelvis. Vertebral body compression deformities tend to have a horizontal linear appearance, whereas rib fractures tend to occur in adjacent ribs, often in a linear pattern. Dual-energy x-ray absorptiometry (DEXA) studies can establish fracture risk in patients with osteoporosis and be used to evaluate the effectiveness of therapy.

REFERENCES

Balseiro J, Brower AC, Ziessman HA. Scintigraphic diagnosis of sacral fractures. *AJR Am J Roentgenol*. 1987;148(1):111–113.
Lyders EM, et al. Imaging and treatment of sacral insufficiency fractures. *AJNR Am J Neuroradiol*. 2010;31(2):201–210.

Case 10

TC-99M HIDA—ACUTE CHOLECYSTITIS

1. a
2. c
3. d
4. a

Discussion

Hepatobiliary iminodiacetic acid (HIDA) radiopharmaceuticals, Tc-99m mebrofenin and Tc-99m disofenin, are extracted and excreted by hepatocytes in a manner similar to bilirubin. Patients should fast for 3 to 4 hours before the examination to avoid a possible false-positive result. Recent meal ingestion may result in gallbladder contraction, preventing entry of the radiotracer. Patients who have fasted for more than 24 hours or are receiving hyperalimentation may benefit from pretreatment with cholecystokinin (CCK) before the study to contract the gallbladder and reduce the likelihood of a false-positive result. CCK will cause the gallbladder to contract and relax the sphincter of Oddi, thereby expelling bile that may have accumulated and that could prevent gallbladder filling.

Nonvisualization of the gallbladder on hepatobiliary scan in the setting of right upper quadrant biliary colic is diagnostic of cystic duct obstruction. Although nonvisualization of the gallbladder at 60 minutes is considered abnormal, delayed imaging of up to 4 hours should be obtained to confirm the diagnosis of acute cholecystitis. Images in this case are from a patient who was allergic to morphine and therefore required delayed imaging (up to 4 hours) for diagnosis.

As 4-hour delayed imaging is not always permissible or optimal in the clinic, morphine may be administered at 60 minutes after visualization of the radiotracer in the bowel. After administration of intravenous morphine, imaging should be continued for an additional 30 minutes. If there is no visualization of the gallbladder, cystic duct obstruction is confirmed. The sensitivity of the examination is greater than 95%, and specificity is greater than 90%.

Acalculous acute cholecystitis is an uncommon condition that may be life threatening. It most commonly occurs in critically ill patients. Early detection and intervention are paramount because the mortality rate is high: approximately 30%. The entity is not caused by a stone in the cystic duct, but rather by inflammatory debris, inspissated bile, and local edema. Some patients develop acute acalculous cholecystitis through direct inflammation of the gallbladder without cystic duct obstruction. The sensitivity of hepatobiliary imaging for acute acalculous cholecystitis is lower than that for calculous cholecystitis because some patients do not have cystic duct obstruction but direct inflammation of the gallbladder. In the setting of high clinical suspicion of a false-negative result (acute cholecystitis but gallbladder filling), sincalide infusion should be considered, because an inflamed gallbladder may not contract normally.

REFERENCES

Choy D, Shi EC, McLean RG, et al. Cholescintigraphy in acute cholecystitis: use of intravenous morphine. *Radiology*. 1984;151(1):203–207.

Ziessman HA. Hepatobiliary scintigraphy–2014. *J Nucl Med*. 2014;55(6):967–975.

Case 11

COLON CANCER—PET/CT

1. b
2. a
3. b
4. b

Discussion

Incidental focal F-18 FDG colonic uptake is a common finding in clinical practice. Diffuse colonic activity without any anatomic abnormality on CT tends to be physiologic or related to medications, such as metformin, and is considered benign. Focal uptake in the bowel is of more concern with regard to an underlying abnormality. However, increased uptake in the ileocecal valve region, compared with the rest of the bowel, is not uncommon, and this is thought to be related to increased lymphoid tissue in this region. Before dismissing focal activity in this region, it is important to look at the anatomic CT images to assess for the presence of a mass. Nonfocal increased activity in the large bowel may be a sign of underlying colitis. In this setting, the anatomic images are likely to demonstrate thickened bowel wall with inflammatory changes in the adjacent fat. Incidental focal uptake in the bowel is seen in 1% of PET/CT images, and over 50% of these lesions have been found to correspond to malignant or premalignant lesions. Thus, these focal regions of colonic uptake with associated CT soft tissue abnormality should be further evaluated with colonoscopy. Although focal diverticulitis may demonstrate increased FDG uptake, subjacent inflammatory changes are expected to be seen on concurrent CT scan.

REFERENCES

Shmidt E, Nehra V, Lowe V, Oxentenko AS. Clinical significance of incidental [18 F] FDG uptake in the gastrointestinal tract on PET/CT imaging: a retrospective cohort study. *BMC Gastroenterol.* 2016;16(1):125.

Treglia G, Calcagni ML, Rufini V, et al. Clinical significance of incidental focal colorectal 18F–fluorodeoxyglucose uptake: our experience and a review of the literature. *Colorectal Dis.* 2012;14(2):174–180.

Case 12

BONE SCAN—OSTEOSARCOMA

1. a
2. d
3. b
4. d

Discussion

Osteosarcoma is the most common malignant bone tumor in children and adolescents. This tumor tends to arise in the metaphyseal region of long bones. The most common sites are distal femur, proximal tibia, and proximal humerus. The example shown in this case is unusual in location—a rib. Tumors may extend into the diaphysis or epiphyses as well as the adjacent soft tissue. MRI is the best modality to evaluate the extent of the primary lesion, especially adjacent soft tissue involvement. These tumors tend to have a classic appearance on plain-film radiography or CT—the starburst appearance, as noted in this case.

Bone scintigraphy is primarily indicated for the evaluation of skip lesions, multicentric osteosarcoma, or primary lesion with metastases. If there are multiple sites of osseous disease, limb amputation is not indicated. CT of the chest is indicated to assess for the presence of pulmonary metastases. However, lung metastases can often be seen on the bone scan. Osteosarcoma is positive on all three bone scan phases. Evaluation for additional sites of disease can be detected on delayed whole-body images. Osteosarcoma lesions are very avid on bone scintigraphy. Bone scan tends to overestimate the extent of primary disease because of the perilesional circulatory changes.

REFERENCES

Choi YY, Kim JY, Yang SO. PET/CT in benign and malignant musculoskeletal tumors and tumor-like conditions. *Semin Musculoskelet Radiol.* 2014;18(2):133–148.

Harrison DJ, Parisi MT, Shulkin BL. The role of 18F-FDG PET/CT in pediatric sarcoma. *Semin In Nucl Med.* 2017;47(3):229–241.

Case 13

THYROID SCAN—COLD NODULE

1. b
2. a
3. b
4. c

Discussion

Iodine-123 (I-123) is the preferred thyroid scintigraphic imaging agent because it is trapped and organified similar to dietary iodine. Tc-99m pertechnetate can also be used for thyroid imaging. It is trapped but not organified by the thyroid. Tc-99m pertechnetate is advantageous in children because of lower radiation dose and higher count rate (shorter imaging time). Tc-99m pertechnetate is administered intravenously, whereas I-123 is given orally. Following I-123 administration, imaging is usually performed at 4 hours.

A pinhole collimator is used for scintigraphic imaging of the thyroid. The lead collimator is shaped like a cone, with a pinhole lead insert at its tip. The collimator magnifies and provides superior resolution compared with a parallel-hole collimator, 2 to 6 mm, depending on the size of the lead pinhole insert.

The differential diagnosis for a photopenic defect in the thyroid gland includes cysts, colloid nodules, focal scarring or inflammation related to thyroiditis, and benign and malignant tumors.

The incidence of thyroid cancer is less than 1% in a hot nodule and 10% to 15% in a cold nodule. Therefore cold nodules must be evaluated with thyroid US. If there are features suggestive of malignancy, such as microcalcifications, a biopsy is recommended.

REFERENCE

Tamhane S, Gharib H. Thyroid nodule update on diagnosis and management. *Clin Diabetes Endocrinol*. 2016;2(1):17.

Case 14

BROWN FAT ON FDG PET/CT

1. b
2. c
3. a
4. c

Discussion

This F-18 FDG PET scan shows increased uptake within brown adipose tissue in the neck and supraclavicular regions and paraspinal regions. In addition to these common sites, it may also be seen in the mediastinum and in the upper abdomen, around the spleen, kidneys, and diaphragm. This case demonstrates classic regions for brown fat activation. F18 FDG uptake in lymphoma would not be expected to demonstrate bilateral, symmetric uptake in the paraspinal regions, as noted in this case.

Hybrid imaging with CT helps identify brown fat activation as opposed to other pathologic causes (e.g., lymphadenopathy).

Findings on maximum-intensity projection (MIP) images should always be confirmed on cross-sectional images. Significant brown fat uptake may obscure abnormal uptake within small lymph nodes. A number of techniques may be employed to reduce the likelihood of brown fat activation before an F18 FDG PET study. These include keeping the patient warm, with a well-heated preparation room and warm blankets, and pretreating the patient with beta blockers or benzodiazepines. This activity tends to occur more frequently and is more prominent in young patients.

REFERENCES

Cohade C, Mourtzikos KA, Wahl RL. USA-Fat: prevalence is related to ambient outdoor temperature—evaluation with 18F-FDG PET/CT. *J Nucl Med*. 2003;44(8):1267–1270.

Truong MT, Erasmus JJ, Munden RF, et al. Focal FDG uptake in mediastinal brown fat mimicking malignancy: a potential pitfall resolved on PET/CT. *Am J Roentgenol*. 2004;183(4):1127–1132.

Case 15

LASIX RENOGRAPHY—RENAL OBSTRUCTION

1. a
2. b
3. a
4. d

Discussion

This patient had right flank pain and a history of renal stones. The renal scan demonstrates decreased perfusion to the right kidney relative to the left kidney (image A). There is delayed cortical uptake and no spontaneous excretion (no collecting system is seen, and the counts curve for the right kidney continues to increase over time). Following the administration of intravenous furosemide (Lasix), there is no excretion of radiotracer (flat curve) compatible with high-grade obstruction (image B). Lasix is not helpful unless it is given with the renal pelvis full of radiotracer. Lasix increases urine flow. The diagnosis could have been made at the end of the initial 30-minute study. This is high-grade obstruction.

Lasix renal scintigraphy is often ordered to evaluate for obstruction. Tc-99m DTPA or mercaptoacetyltriglycine (MAG3) may be used to perform the study. However, in patients with compromised renal function, MAG3 is preferred. The mechanism of Tc-99m MAG3 is tubular uptake that represents 80% of renal function. The mechanism of uptake for Tc-99m DTPA is glomerular function, which represents 10% to 20% of renal function. Hydration before imaging should be routine, intravenously for children and orally for adolescents and adults. In the setting of dehydration, excretion of radiotracer may be delayed (pseudo-obstruction). In the setting of a neurogenic bladder or bladder outlet obstruction, placement of a Foley catheter should be considered to relieve retrograde pressure that may simulate obstruction on scintigraphy. This should be routine in infants and children.

In patients with a history of hydronephrosis, the clinical question is whether this is caused by obstruction. Lasix is administered when the collecting system has filled. Lasix works by blocking the tubular reabsorption of sodium, chloride, and water, resulting in increased diuresis in a nonobstructed kidney. Good washout excludes obstruction. No or poor washout is consistent with obstruction. A half-time of emptying (t½) is calculated. Generally, there is no obstruction if the t½ is less than 10 minutes and obstructed if the t½ is greater than 20. It is interpreted as an indeterminate study between these two values. Care must be taken to ensure that the correct region of interest (i.e., the collecting system) has been drawn.

REFERENCES

Howman-Giles R, Uren R, Roy LP, Filmer RB. Volume expansion diuretic renal scan in urinary tract obstruction. *J Nucl Med.* 1987;28(5):824–828.

Perez-Brayfield MR, Kirsch AJ, Jones RA, Grattan-Smith JD. A prospective study comparing ultrasound, nuclear scintigraphy and dynamic contrast enhanced magnetic resonance imaging in the evaluation of hydronephrosis. *J Urol.* 2003;170(4):1330–1334.

Case 16

TC-99M RBC—GI BLEED–DESCENDING/PROXIMAL SIGMOID BLEED

1. c
2. a
3. a
4. c

Discussion

Gastrointestinal (GI) bleeding studies are performed to localize the site of an active lower GI bleed so that effective therapy can be performed. This study demonstrates increased uptake in the left lower quadrant compatible with left descending/proximal sigmoid colon bleed. The findings meet all the criteria for diagnosis of an active bleed—the uptake conforms to the bowel contour, moves retrograde or antegrade over time, and increases in intensity over time.

Because the radiopharmaceutical remains in the blood pool during the length of the study, imaging can be performed up to 24 hours. Tc-99m binds to the beta chain of the hemoglobin molecule. There are three methods for labeling: in vitro, modified in vivo (vitro), and in vivo. The in vitro method has the highest labeling efficiency of greater than 90%. The organs receiving the highest radiation dose (critical organs) for this study are the spleen and the myocardial wall.

Most GI bleeds will be visualized within 90 minutes of imaging. Increased gastric and thyroid uptake suggests that there was poor labeling (free pertechnetate). GI bleeding scans are very sensitive for detecting small bleeds (0.1 mL/min) compared with contrast angiography (1 mL/min). Bleeding scans allow for targeted therapy in the interventional suite. The sooner that the study is done after arrival in the emergency room or admission, the higher the likelihood of obtaining a positive result on the bleeding scan study.

REFERENCES

Dam HQ, Brandon DC, Grantham VV, et al. The SNMMI procedure standard/EANM practice guideline for gastrointestinal bleeding scintigraphy. *J Nucl Med Technol.* 2014;42(4):308–317.

Grady E. Gastrointestinal bleeding scintigraphy in the early 21st century. *J Nucl Med.* 2016;57(2):252–259.

Case 17

BONE SCAN—PAGET'S DISEASE

1. d
2. a
3. b
4. b

Discussion

This study demonstrates increased radiotracer uptake in the left humerus (extending from the epiphysis) and in a vertebral body at the thoracolumbar junction. The abnormality in the spine has a "Mickey Mouse" appearance highly suggestive of Paget's disease. Paget's disease is another entity that may have a three-phase positive bone scan. However, the three-phase study is rarely performed or needed, and the diagnosis is often made incidentally, as in this case.

Paget's disease is usually asymptomatic. Bone pain or an elevated alkaline phosphatase (more common) is often the reason for referral for the evaluation of underlying Paget's disease. The scintigraphic pattern is typically intense uptake involving most of a bone. The main differential of this scan is metastatic disease versus Paget's disease. Radiographic correlation is necessary.

Paget's disease is a chronic benign disease in the elderly and has an unknown etiology. The pelvis is the most common bone involved, followed by the spine, skull, femur, scapula, tibia, and humerus.

The uptake in both the humerus and spine in this patient are very characteristic for Paget's disease. The radiographic appearance is classically described as having three phases: lytic, mixed lytic/sclerotic, and sclerotic. X-ray findings are characterized by coarsened trabecula and expanded bone. Lesions tend to extend to the end of long bones. Twenty percent of lesions are monostotic. A complication of this disease is high-output congestive heart failure related to increased blood flow to the abnormal bone.

REFERENCES

Ralsoton SH. Paget's disease of bone. *The N Engl J Med.* 2013;368(7):644–650.

Smith SE, Murphey MD, Motamedi K, Mulligan ME, Resnik CS, Gannon FH. Radiologic spectrum of Paget disease of bone and its complications with pathologic correlation. *Radiographics.* 2002;22(5):1191–1216.

Theodorou DJ, Stavroula JT, Kabitsubata Y. Imaging of Paget disease of bone and its musculoskeletal complications: review. *AJR.* 2011;196(suppl 6):S64–S75.

Case 18

F-18 FDG PET/CT—LYMPHOMA

1. d
2. d
3. a
4. c

Discussion

This F-18 FDG PET scan demonstrates abnormal FDG activity throughout the neck, chest, and abdomen, most compatible with a diagnosis of lymphoma. The axial fused and CT images demonstrate that this activity localizes to a lymph node conglomeration within the abdomen, thus excluding the diagnosis of brown fat. The heterogeneous, nonuniform uptake on the MIP images should also sway against the diagnosis of brown fat.

There are many types of lymphomas requiring different therapies, depending on histology, immunohistochemical profile, and cytogenetic profile. The Ann Arbor staging classification system may be applied to both Hodgkin's lymphoma and non-Hodgkin's lymphoma (NHL). There are four stages: I: single lymph node group; II: more than one lymph node group on one side of the diaphragm; III: lymph node groups above and below the diaphragm; and IV: noncontiguous extranodal involvement, including bone marrow, lungs, and the liver. This case demonstrates nodal disease above and below the diaphragm. Stage IV was not an option, obviating the need to infer whether some of the FDG-avid lesions were extranodal or not.

F-18 FDG PET/CT plays an important role in the staging and treatment response assessment of FDG-avid lymphomas. Low-grade lymphomas, in particular gastrointestinal lymphomas, may not be FDG avid, and this limits the utility of this technique. A baseline scan should be acquired so that subsequent interim and follow-up scans can provide the most information regarding response to therapy. Also, extranodal disease, in particular bone marrow disease, is often better appreciated on F-18 FDG PET/CT compared with conventional CT imaging. No definite thresholds for change in standardized uptake value (SUV) measurements have been established to assess whether the response to therapy is complete or partial. CT criteria alone, using Response Evaluation Criteria in Solid Tumors (RECIST) measurements, may be used in isolation to evaluate for residual or recurrent disease in FDG-avid lymphomas.

The Lugano classification was established by a consensus group of experts to standardize response assessment and reporting for lymphomas. This classification is a five-point system based on qualitative analysis. A Lugano score of 1 to 3 is compatible with complete metabolic response. The reference points are activity in the liver and mediastinal blood pool. A score of 3 demonstrates activity similar to that of the liver, whereas scores of 1 and 2 demonstrate "no activity" and "activity similar to blood pool," respectively. Lugano scores of 4 and 5 are compatible with partial response and no response. A score of 4 is compatible with activity slightly greater than that of the liver, whereas a score of 5 is compatible with activity much greater than that of the liver. No numerical SUV thresholds have been established. Progressive disease is diagnosed in the setting of new FDG-avid disease and/or increased activity in Lugano 4/5 disease that has increased from baseline.

REFERENCES

Cheson BD, Fisher RI, Barrington SF, et al. Recommendations for initial evaluation, staging, and response assessment of Hodgkin and non-Hodgkin lymphoma: the Lugano classification. *J Clin Oncol*. 2014;32(27):3059–3067.

Johnson SA, Kumar A, Matasar MJ, Schöder H, Rademaker J. Imaging for staging and response assessment in lymphoma. *Radiology*. 2015;276(2): 323–338.

Case 19

TC-99M HIDA—CHRONIC ACALCULOUS CHOLECYSTITIS

1. b
2. b
3. b
4. c

Discussion

Chronic cholecystitis may be characterized as calculous or acalculous. Patients with calculous chronic cholecystitis are infrequently evaluated with scintigraphy, because the presence of gallstones is established with US and the patients undergo surgery. However, patients with acalculous cholecystitis are frequently referred for a sincalide (CCK) hepatobiliary scan to calculate the gallbladder ejection fraction (GBEF). These patients typically present with recurrent biliary colic similar to patients with calculous chronic cholecystitis. An abnormal sincalide cholescintigraphy study can identify patients who likely have the disease and can obtain symptomatic relief after surgical removal of the gallbladder. The recommended sincalide dose is 0.02 µg/kg infused over 60 minutes after the visualization of the gallbladder. A consensus paper has recommended a standard infusion period of 60 minutes. Shorter infusion times may induce abdominal cramping, nausea, and/or vomiting and result in a more variable and unpredictable GBEF response. The lower threshold of normal for the GBEF is 38%.

REFERENCES

DiBaise John K, et al. Cholecystokinin-cholescintigraphy in adults: consensus recommendations of an interdisciplinary panel. *Clin Gastroenterol Hepatol*. 2011;9(5):376–384.

Ziessman HA, Tulchinsky M, Lavely WC, et al. Sincalide-stimulated cholescintigraphy: a multicenter investigation to determine optimal infusion methodology and gallbladder ejection fraction normal values. *J Nucl Med*. 2010;51(2):277–281.

Case 20

F-18 FDG PET/CT—LUNG CANCER

1. a
2. a
3. a
4. d

Discussion

This case demonstrates a single lesion in the right upper lobe without evidence of F-18 FDG-avid lymphadenopathy in the mediastinum or elsewhere. The stage of this 3-cm lesion without evidence of nodal disease is Ia. Stage IIIb includes contralateral nodal disease or supraclavicular nodal disease. Patients with stage IIIb disease are thought to be unresectable at presentation. Neoadjuvant chemotherapy and radiation may downgrade the staging and allow for resection.

Lung cancer is one of the most common cancer in both women and men and a leading cause of cancer-related deaths. F-18 FDG PET/CT plays a role in the evaluation of pulmonary nodules, staging of lung cancer as well as therapy assessment. Staging of lung cancer follows the TNM (tumor–node–metastasis) staging system. Post-therapy assessment of lung cancer can be difficult because of increased radiotracer uptake indefinitely after radiation. Serial imaging may help in the assessment of recurrence, which can be expected to demonstrate a more focal area of increased uptake that persists or increases over time. FDG PET/CT plays a significant role in staging because it may detect distant metastases that may be occult on clinical examination and other imaging studies.

REFERENCES

American Cancer Society. Cancer Facts & Figure 2013. Atlanta, GA: American Cancer Society; 2013. Available from http://www.cancer.org/research/cancerfactsfigures/cancerfactsfigures/cancer-facts-figures-2013. Accessed on Nov 21, 2013.

American NCCN Clinical Practice Guidelines in Oncology – Non-small cell lung cancer v4.2017 Jan 18, 2017.

Case 21

QUALITY CONTROL FLOOD IMAGE

1. b
2. a
3. a
4. b

Discussion

This is a normal flood source image. Quality control in nuclear medicine is paramount and is thus performed at required specified intervals on gamma cameras. This image is a uniformity flood image, which must be performed daily. The purpose is to evaluate the consistency of response of a gamma camera to a uniform flux of radiation. Although the source may be contained liquid with any radionuclide imaged with a gamma camera, most centers utilize a solid, sealed source of cobalt-57 (Co-57; keV 122). This test is performed before any clinical studies are performed. Between 5 million and 20 million counts are acquired, and the image is assessed qualitatively for any defects or irregularity. If the image is not homogeneous and uniform, the cause must be determined, often requiring manufacturer service.

REFERENCE

Murphy PH. Acceptance testing and quality control of gamma cameras, including SPECT. *J Nucl Med*. 1987;28(7):1221–1227.

Case 22

SUPERSCAN—RENAL FAILURE

1. d
2. b
3. a
4. b

Discussion

Some metabolic conditions are associated with increased osseous uptake of radiotracer on bone scintigraphy (e.g., renal osteodystrophy, osteomalacia, hypervitaminosis D, and hyperparathyroidism). In patients with these conditions, the typical findings on scintigraphy include diffusely increased uptake in the axial skeleton, skull, mandible, and sternum ("tie" pattern) and significantly reduced or absent soft tissue and renal activity. The term often used for this pattern of uptake is *superscan* because it appears to be of superior quality. Soft tissue and kidneys show minimal activity as a result of the high bone uptake, leaving less activity in the soft tissue and for renal clearance, but the appearance is also caused by a scaling factor.

A delay in imaging results in less renal and soft tissue activity because of background and renal clearance. Regional or focal increased uptake can be seen in osteomalacia (pseudofractures), Paget's disease, and osteoporosis (compression fractures).

In renal failure, secondary hyperparathyroidism occurs as a result of hypocalcemia. With long-standing renal dysfunction, one or more parathyroid gland(s) may become autonomous, producing hypercalcemia (tertiary hyperparathyroidism). A superscan may be seen in this setting.

Diffuse metastatic disease may have a similar appearance as a result of diffuse metabolic bone disease. However, the superscan resulting from metastatic disease is usually associated with some regional variability and focal uptake. Additionally, intense uptake in the skull, as seen in this patient, is more characteristic of metabolic bone diseases, such as secondary hyperparathyroidism. Granulocyte colony-stimulating factor (GCSF) and metformin have no effect on the bone scan. This patient had renal failure. Uptake in the right axilla is an A-V shunt for dialysis.

REFERENCES

Grellier J-F, Lussato D, Queneau M, et al. Secondary hyperparathyroidism with "superscan-like" hypermetabolic FDG PET/CT pattern. *Clin Nucl Med.* 2015;40(11):888–889.

Kulkarni M, Soni A, Shetkar, et al. Coexistent superscan and Lincoln sign on bone scintigraphy. *Clin Nucl Med.* 2017;42(8):630–632.

Love C, Din AS, Tomas MB, Kalapparambath TP, Palestro CJ. Radionuclide bone imaging: an illustrative review. *Radiographics.* 2003;23(2): 341–358.

Case 23

MYOCARDIAL PERFUSION STUDY—CARDIAC ISCHEMIA

1. a
2. d
3. b
4. a

Discussion

Radionuclide myocardial stress perfusion studies are a noninvasive method to assess myocardial perfusion and function, allowing the cardiologist to risk-stratify the patient. The finding on this study is a stress-induced myocardial perfusion defect involving the inferior wall of the heart. The rest study is normal. This is consistent with ischemia of the inferior wall, which is supplied by the right coronary artery. A myocardial infarction would show reduced perfusion at stress and rest. Tc-99m sestamibi delivery to the myocardium depends on blood flow and retention within the cell. The latter requires viable myocardium. The radiopharmaceutical, Tc-99m sestamibi, is normally retained in the myocardial cell in the region of mitochondria. A pharmacologic stress test is only performed when the patient cannot exercise to provide valuable clinical information to the cardiologist's assessment of the patient. The resulting images from exercise and pharmacologic stress tests are similar, although the mechanisms are different. With exercise, stress-induced ischemia is characterized by relatively reduced blood flow, which normalizes at rest. The pharmacologic stress agents cause coronary vasodilatation. Stenotic vessels cannot dilate to the extent that nonstenotic vessels can, explaining the differential flow seen. The two methods of stress provide similar information on the status of coronary blood flow and have similar accuracy.

REFERENCES

Muzaffar R, Raslan O, Ahmed F, et al. Incidental findings on myocardial perfusion SPECT images. *J Nucl Med Technol*. 2017;45(3):175–180.

Travin MI. Pitfalls and limitations of radionuclide and hybrid cardiac imaging. *Semin Nucl Med*. 2015;45(5):392–410.

Case 24

PARATHYROID SCINTIGRAPHY—ADENOMA

1. d
2. b
3. a
4. d

Discussion

This is a planar Tc-99m sestamibi study for localization of a para-thyroid adenoma or hyperplasia. The study shows abnormal radio-tracer accumulation inferior to the left thyroid gland, increasing on the delayed images, consistent with a parathyroid adenoma.

Parathyroid hormone (PTH) regulates calcium and phospho-rous homeostasis by acting on bone, the small intestine, and the renal system. Primary hyperparathyroidism is usually caused by a single autonomous, hyperfunctioning parathyroid adenoma (85%). Hyperplasia (10%–15%) and parathyroid carcinoma (<1%) are less common. Today, most patients with hyperparathyroidism are detected incidentally with an elevated serum calcium on routine blood studies. Parathyroid adenomas may occur in ectopic locations, for example, adjacent to the carotid bifurcations, inferior mediasti-num, and tracheoesophageal groove. The scan plays a pivotal role for the surgeon because with this information, most parathyroid adenomas can be removed with a minimally invasive approach.

Localization of parathyroid adenomas with Tc-99m sestamibi, the same agent as used for myocardial perfusion scintigraphy, is dependent on the high cellularity of adenomas. The radiotracer is retained in close proximity to mitochondria.

A variety of imaging methodologies are used at different clinics. Planar imaging is often performed; however, SPECT and SPECT/CT are increasingly utilized because of improved localization. Early (10 minutes) and delayed (2 hours) imaging is common. Tc-99m sestamibi is taken up by the thyroid and para-thyroid but clears from the thyroid faster than the hyperfunction-ing parathyroid adenoma so that delayed imaging in the majority of cases will show only the parathyroid adenoma.

Alternatively, a dual radiotracer protocol can be obtained, wherein a thyroid-only radiotracer, either I-123 or Tc-99m pertechnetate, is administered and the thyroid planar image is subtracted from the parathyroid Tc-99m sestamibi scan. The subtracted image will show the parathyroid adenoma.

Tc-99m sestamibi has a higher accuracy for detection com-pared with US, CT, or MRI. The most common cause for a false-negative result is small size. False-positive results may occur in the setting of thyroid adenoma and multinodular goiter. Sensi-tivity for identifying a parathyroid adenoma is about 90% once they reach a size of 300 mg or larger. Patients with four-gland hyperplasia have a lower sensitivity for detection.

REFERENCES

Lavely WC, Goetze S, Friedman KP, et al. Comparison of SPECT/CT, SPECT, and planar imaging with single- and dual-phase 99mTc-ses-tamibi parathyroid scintigraphy. *J Nucl Med.* 2007;48(7):1084–1089.

Nguyen BD. Parathyroid imaging with Tc-99m sestamibi planar and SPECT scintigraphy. *Radiographics.* 1999;19(3):601–614.

Case 25

THYROID TOXIC ADENOMA

1. c
2. b
3. b
4. b

Discussion

A hot nodule is defined as a palpable or ultrasonographically confirmed nodule that demonstrates increased radiotracer uptake on an I-123 scan. The nodule has autonomous function, whereas the normal adjacent thyroid responds to the normal thyroid/pituitary feedback. An autonomously functioning hot nodule will suppress the remaining gland if it is large enough (>2.5 cm) to produce enough T_4/T_3 to suppress TSH (as seen in this case). Thus, a small hot autonomous nodule may not produce overt hyperthyroidism, although, with time, it will likely grow and produce thyrotoxicosis. In the interim, there may be partial suppression of the thyroid gland, at which time patients may be symptomatic. Hot nodules tend to have uptake in the normal or high normal range, considerably lower than with Graves' disease. Some nodules that appear "hot" on Tc-99m pertechnetate scans may be photopenic on I-123 scans and thus are not truly autonomous hot nodules. An I-123 scan is necessary to confirm the presence of an autonomous functioning nodule. The linear dash marking on the image is a ruler that allows for size estimation of the nodule as well as the gland, if visualized. This may be useful for dose calculation.

Compared with Graves' disease, toxic nodules are more resistant to I-131 therapy. Hence, the dose of I-131 therapy is higher than that commonly used for Graves' disease. The administered doses typically range from 25 to 30 mCi. Because the surrounding thyroid gland is suppressed, it does not take up the I-131 so that after therapy, most patients become euthyroid as the suppressed gland recovers function. These patients are less likely to develop hypothyroidism with time as seen with patients with Graves' disease treated with I-131.

REFERENCES

Ferrari C, Reschini E, Paracchi A. Treatment of the autonomous thyroid nodule: a review. *Eur J Endocrinol*. 1996;135(4):383–390.

Ross DS, Burch HB, Cooper DS, et al. 2016 American thyroid association guidelines for diagnosis and management of hyperthyroidism and other causes of thyrotoxicosis. *Thyroid*. 2016;26(10):1343–1421.

Case 26

BONE SCAN—COLON UPTAKE

1. d
2. b
3. a
4. c

Discussion

If a patient has received a radionuclide study within 24 hours of a second radionuclide examination, it is prudent to obtain an image before injecting the second radiopharmaceutical for nuclear medicine examination. That was not done in this case, and luckily the colon uptake only obscures a minimal portion of the bone. The 6-hour half-life of Tc-99m allows for easy determination of residual activity at a certain time after injection. This can be done by simple calculation—for example, at 6 hours after injection, half of the activity will remain, and at 12 hours, another half of the activity will decay, and so on. Alternatively, there are decay calculators or decay correction factors that can easily be looked up for an individual radionuclide.

Tc-99m MDP can be prepared from a kit. The kit contains stannous ion stabilizers, and MDP. The stannous ion acts as a reduction agent allowing the Tc-99m to bind to the MDP molecule. If the kit is exposed to air, incomplete labeling may occur because of oxidation of the stannous ion.

Other possible explanations for intestinal visualization on a bone scan include necrotizing enterocolitis, inflammatory conditions, prior urinary diversion surgery, GI bleeding, systemic amyloidosis, and protein-losing enteropathy. Because this patients had no clinical symptoms, diverticulitis is much less likely. Besides colonic uptake, this bone scan looks appropriate making radiolabeling error unlikely. Metformin therapy has no impact on bone scan imaging.

REFERENCES

Kim SH, Song BI, Won KS. Colon visualization on (99m) Tc-HDP whole body bone scan due to sigmoid colon cancer-related enterovesical fistula. *Clin Nucl Med*. 2015;40(8):658–659.

Uzuner O, Ziessman HA. Protein-losing enteropathy detected by T-99m-MDP abdominal scintigraphy. *Pediatr Radiol*. 2008;38(10):1122–1124.

Case 27

FDG PET—METFORMIN

1. a
2. d
3. b
4. a

Discussion

When interpreting F-18 FDG PET/CT images, it is important to be aware of possible false-positive findings. Patients being treated with metformin for type 2 diabetes will often demonstrate increased activity in the large bowel wall (sometimes also in the small bowel wall). Metformin is an oral biguanide used for type 2 diabetes. The high bowel activity limits evaluation by F-18 FDG PET/CT for bowel pathology. However, the CT portion should reassure one that there is no inflammatory disease. Studies have shown that discontinuing the drug 2 days before the examination reduces bowel uptake. The patient should be NPO (nothing by mouth) at least 4 to 6 hours before the examination to reduce muscle and cardiac uptake and maximize tumor uptake. Long-acting insulin should be withheld for 12 hours before the study for the same reason. The uptake seen on this MIP image in the parotids is within normal variation. Uptake is also seen in the shoulders and knees, consistent with an inflammatory component of arthritis. The high brain uptake is normal physiologic uptake and the reason for lowered sensitivity for detection of brain metastases.

REFERENCES

Oh JR, Song HC, Chong A, et al. Impact of medication discontinuation on increased intestinal FDG accumulation in diabetic patients treated with metformin. *AJR Am J Roentgenol*. 2010;195(6):1404–1410.

Shreve PD, Anzai Y, Wahl RL. Pitfalls in oncologic diagnosis with FDG PET imaging: physiologic and benign variants. *Radiographics*. 1999;19(1):61–77.

Case 28

RADIOACTIVE DECAY

1. d
2. c
3. c
4. b

Discussion

Radioactive decay is the process by which unstable nuclides transform themselves into more stable entities by releasing energy. We take advantage of this process in nuclear medicine. Several modes of radioactive decay play a role in imaging and treating patients.

The most common are beta decay, positron decay, electron capture, isomeric transition, and alpha decay.

Alpha decay occurs by emitting an alpha particle that consists of two neutrons and two protons. This mode of decay is heavily ionizing and therefore plays a role in therapy. Alpha particles tend to deposit most of their energy over short distances, fraction of a millimeter. Radium-223 (Ra-223) therapy for prostate cancer metastatic to bones is an example.

Beta decay is another mode resulting in significant ionizing radiation. Common radionuclides in nuclear medicine that undergo this type of decay include I-131 and molybdenum-99 (Mo-99).

In positron decay (proton rich), a positively charged beta particle is emitted from the nucleus. This will lead to annihilation resulting in the production of two 511-keV photons, the basis for PET imaging. The transition energy for this process to occur must be equal to or be greater than 1022 keV (two 511-keV photons).

Electron capture is an additional mode by which proton-rich radionuclides undergo decay. In this setting, an inner shell electron is absorbed into the nucleus resulting in an increase of neutrons by 1. No energy threshold is necessary for this to occur. Thallium-201 (The-201), gallium-67 (Ga-67), I-123, and In-111 undergo electron capture.

The most commonly used radionuclide in the nuclear medicine clinic is Tc-99m. Tc-99 undergoes isomeric transition, resulting in no change in atomic number but decrease in energy level with the emission of a gamma photon.

REFERENCE

Ziessman HA, O'Malley JP, Thrall JH. *Nuclear Medicine: The Requisites E-Book*. Elsevier Health Sciences; 2013.

Case 29

TC-99M DMSA—ACUTE PYELONEPHRITIS

1. b
2. c
3. a
4. b

Discussion

Tc-99m DMSA (dimercaptosuccinic acid) is the most sensitive imaging method for the diagnosis of acute pyelonephritis and renal scarring. Binding of 40% to 50% of the radiopharmaceutical to the proximal tubules of the renal cortex and glomerular filtration of the remaining tracer allows for high-resolution planar and/or SPECT images by 2 hours after injection. This case demonstrates a focal defect in the upper pole of the left kidney resolving at 6 months, which is consistent with pyelonephritis. Acute pyelonephritis produces renal tubular dysfunction and results in reduced cortical uptake. In some cases, it may be difficult to differentiate renal scarring from focal infection. Secondary signs, such as a small kidney, decreased cortical thickness, renal distortion at the site of the scar, and a wedge-shaped defect, suggest underlying scarring, whereas acute pyelonephritis may be seen with normal renal contour but reduced uptake. Two such regions are seen initially in the left upper and lower pole. Defects associated with acute pyelonephritis may resolve over time in about 40% of cases. Six-month follow-up imaging allows for adequate time for recovery. Any abnormality that persists for greater than 6 months should be considered to represent a scar. Planar imaging with a pinhole collimator is commonly used to improve resolution over a parallel-hole collimator. SPECT is optional but may require sedation in small children.

REFERENCES

Rushton HG, Majd M. Dimercaptosuccinic acid renal scintigraphy for the evaluation of pyelonephritis and scarring: a review of experimental and clinical studies. *J Urol*. 1992;148(5):1726–1732.

Zaki M, Badawi M, Al Mutari G, Ramadan D, Rahman MA. Acute pyelonephritis and renal scarring in Kuwaiti children: a follow-up study using 99mTc DMSA renal scintigraphy. *Pediatr Nephrol*. 2005;20(8):1116–1119.

Case 30

MECKEL'S SCAN

1. d
2. a
3. b
4. a

Discussion

This case shows focal radiotracer accumulation in an unexpected and somewhat unusual location, superior to the bladder. Uptake in Meckel's diverticulum is most commonly seen in the right lower quadrant. The study is consistent with heterotopic gastric mucosa, likely in a Meckel's diverticulum.

The most common anomaly of the gastrointestinal system is Meckel's diverticulum. It is caused by failure of the omphalomesenteric duct to close. This true diverticulum arises from the antimesenteric side of the distal small bowel and measures about 2 to 3 cm. It most commonly occurs in young children; however, it has been reported in older children and rarely in adults. The most common complication is ulceration of the diverticulum or the adjacent small bowel resulting in bleeding and possible perforation. Approximately 10% to 30% Meckel's diverticula contain gastric mucosa. Meckel's diverticula that bleed have gastric mucosa.

Tc-99m pertechnetate is taken up by the gastric mucosa. Patients are typically pretreated for the study with cimetidine or other histamine 2 (H_2) receptor antagonist, which inhibits release of the radiotracer from the gastric mucosa. Uptake in the diverticulum occurs at the same time as gastric uptake. The most common reason for a false-positive result is radiotracer in the renal pelvis or ureter. However, there is a long list of reported false-positive results, including inflammatory bowel disease and duplication cysts that contain gastric mucosa, but they are uncommon.

REFERENCES

Emamian SA, Shalaby-Rana E, Majd M. The spectrum of heterotopic gastric mucosa in children detected by Tc-99m pertechnetate scintigraphy. *Clin Nucl Med.* 2001;2001(26):529–535.

Spottswood SE, Pfluger T, Bartold SP, et al. SNMMI and EANM practice guideline for Meckel's diverticulum scintigraphy. *J Nucl Med Technol.* 2014;42(3):163–169.

Case 31

CYSTOGRAPHY—VESICOURETERAL REFLUX

1. d
2. a
3. b
4. b

Discussion

Vesicoureteral reflux (VUR) is caused by failure of the uretero-vesical valve. The normal ureter courses through the bladder wall obliquely so that when the bladder fills with urine, the valve passively closes to prevent reflux. VUR occurs in approximately 1% to 2 % of the pediatric population. In the setting of pyelonephritis, the occurrence of reflux is approximately 40%. In up to 80% of patients, the reflux will resolve spontaneously as the child grows and the ureter elongates. The likelihood of renal damage is directly related to the grade of the reflux.

There are two common methods for evaluation of VUR: radionuclide cystography and voiding cystourethrography (VCUG; fluoroscopic procedure). The radionuclide procedure is more sensitive for the detection of reflux (detects volumes of 1 mL) and results in significantly less radiation exposure.

Radionuclide cystography has three components:
1. Continuous imaging during bladder filling
2. Continuous imaging during micturition
3. Postvoid images

Tc-99m sulfur colloid or Tc-99m DTPA can be used for the study. A solution of 1 mCi radiotracer in 500 mL of saline is adequate.

In contrast to VCUG grading, cystography grading has three levels:

Grade 1: activity limited to the ureter (VCUG grade I)
Grade 2: activity reaching the collecting system with none or minimal activity in ureter (VCUG grades II and III)
Grade 3: activity reaching a dilated collecting system and tortuous ureter (VCUG grades IV and V)

This case demonstrates bilateral reflux, left greater than right.

The reflux on the left extends to the renal pelvis, hence a scintigraphic grade of 2.

REFERENCES

Joaquim AI, deGodoy MF, Burdmann EA. Cyclic direct radionuclide cystography in the diagnosis and characterization of vesicoureteral reflux in children and adults. *Clin Nucl Med.* 2015;40(8):627–631.

Piepsz A, Ham HR. Pediatric applications of renal nuclear medicine. *Semin Nucl Med.* 200; 36(1):16–35.

Case 32

F-18 FDG PET—GCSF

1. a
2. c
3. b
4. a

Discussion

This case demonstrates increased radiotracer uptake throughout the visualized bone marrow/osseous structures, consistent with GCSF treatment–related changes. In certain patients, evaluation of the bone marrow may be somewhat limited by physiologic response to therapy. Specifically, administration of GCSF may result in diffuse, increased tracer uptake in bone marrow. GCSF is a hematopoietic cytokine that is used to treat anemia or chemotherapy-induced neutropenia. This finding is most often readily differentiated from diffuse metastatic disease, which has a more heterogeneous appearance, with areas of focal uptake above background. Concurrent CT images may also assist in differentiating the two because osseous lesions may be seen as abnormalities on CT. If clinically possible, follow-up scanning should be delayed until the effect of the therapy has subsided. Recent physical activity, failure to fast, or trauma would not be expected to result in diffusely increased FDG uptake in the bony structures.

REFERENCES

Hanaoka K, et al. Fluorodeoxyglucose uptake in the bone marrow after granulocyte colony-stimulating factor administration in patients with non-Hodgkin's lymphoma. *Nucl Med Commun*. 2011;32(8):678–683.

Kazama T, et al. Effect of colony-stimulating factor and conventional- or high-dose chemotherapy on FDG uptake in bone marrow. *Eur J Nucl Med Mol Imaging*. 2005;32(12):1406–1411.

Case 33

STAR EFFECT

1. b
2. a
3. b
4. a

Discussion

After I-131 therapy for thyroid cancer, imaging is often obtained 1 week later. Approximately 10% of patients will have metastases not detected on the I-123 scan before therapy. On the post-therapy scan, it is not uncommon to see intense uptake in the thyroid bed in this pattern of a "star artifact." This is caused by the high-energy I-131 photons that penetrate the hexagonal collimator lead septa (six-pointed star). The clinical problem with this artifact is that it can obscure nodal or upper mediastinal disease. Neither lead attenuation nor SPECT can help. A medium- or high-energy pinhole collimator could solve this problem because it has no septa. Today, most departments have only low-energy collimators, which would produce considerable high-energy scatter artifact. The liver is routinely seen on post-therapy scans because of the normal metabolism of radiolabeled thyroid hormone.

REFERENCE

Ziessman HA, O'Malley JP, Thrall JH. *Nuclear Medicine: The Requisites E-Book*. Elsevier Health Sciences; 2013.

Case 34

HIDA—BILIARY ATRESIA

1. a
2. d
3. b
4. a

Discussion

Neonatal hepatitis and biliary atresia have similar clinical presentations. Early diagnosis is essential because the timing of surgery is critical to the outcome. The best outcome occurs when surgery for biliary atresia is performed within the first 3 months of life. The pathophysiology of biliary atresia includes progressive sclerosing cholangitis of the extrahepatic biliary tree with periportal fibrosis. There is relative paucity or absence of the major biliary ducts. This may lead to cirrhosis, if not corrected. The Kasai procedure is performed initially, followed by liver transplantation. In the Kasai procedure, the extrahepatic ducts are removed, after which hepatoportoenterostomy is performed.

Hepatobiliary scintigraphy has high sensitivity (97%) but somewhat lower specificity. There are other conditions that may mimic biliary atresia on scintigraphy. The most common one is neonatal hepatitis. The biliary tree and bowel are not visualized over 24-hour imaging in both conditions (as seen in this case). Pretreatment with phenobarbital increases the sensitivity of this study by activating the liver enzymes. The serum phenobarbital level should be in the therapeutic range before imaging. This will significantly improve specificity. However, even with preadministration of phenobarbital, false-positive results do occur in the setting of neonatal hepatitis.

REFERENCES

Kwatra N, et al. Phenobarbital-enhanced hepatobiliary scintigraphy in the diagnosis of biliary atresia: two decades of experience at a tertiary center. *Pediatr Radiol*. 2013;43(10):1365–1375.

Nadel HR. Hepatobiliary scintigraphy in children. *Semin Nucl Med*. 1991;26(1):25–42.

Case 35

BONE SCAN—HORSESHOE KIDNEY

1. c
2. a
3. b
4. a

Discussion

In addition to evaluating the skeletal structures for abnormalities on bone scintigraphy, it is important to always take note of soft tissues and the kidneys because it may help identify important abnormalities. This case demonstrates the presence of a horseshoe kidney. It is normal to see activity within the renal system on bone scans. It is important to include the renal system in the search pattern because obstructive disease or congenital anomalies may be first detected on bone scans obtained for other indications. Horseshoe kidney is a congenital entity affecting 1 per 600 persons. The inferior poles are fused, and this is referred to as the *isthmus*. Sometimes, the point of connection of the two kidneys does not take up the tracer. However, the kidneys are oriented abnormally, with the inferior poles facing each other.

The isthmus is located below the origin of the internal mesenteric artery, thus preventing ascent of the horseshoe kidney. These patients are at increased risk for development of renal stones, infections, obstruction, and renal neoplasia, including Wilms' tumor and transitional cell carcinoma.

This anomaly often goes undetected, and thus it is important to note this in bone scintigraphy reports.

Uptake in the neck in this patient is caused by thyroid cartilage calcification, often seen in elderly patients. Peak radiotracer uptake in bone on a bone scan is at 1 hour. However, imaging is performed at 3 hours to provide time for background clearance, resulting in increased bone-to-soft tissue uptake and superior image quality.

REFERENCES

Mendichovszky I, Solar BT, Smeulders N, et al. Nuclear medicine in pedia-tric nephro-urology: an overview. *Semin Nucl Med*. 2017;47(3):204–228.

Natsis K, Piagkou M, Skotsimara A, Protogerou V, Tsitouridis I, Skandalakis P. Horseshoe kidney: a review of anatomy and pathology. *Surg Radiol Anat*. 2014;36(6):517–526.

Case 36

F-18 FDG PET—HEAD AND NECK CANCER

1. d
2. b
3. a
4. c

Discussion

This scan demonstrates a right tongue base lesion with ipsilateral metastatic level II adenopathy.

Squamous cell cancer of the tongue base has a poor prognosis, so staging is paramount when devising a treatment plan to avoid unnecessary procedures. Head and neck cancer is the sixth most common cancer worldwide. The majority of these cancers are squamous cell cancers. Most patients present with locally advanced disease. F-18 FDG PET/CT is useful in staging, post-treatment evaluation, and recurrence assessment. Staging of head and neck cancer is based on the TNM system. The presence of metastatic nodes is predictive of a poor outcome.

Synchronous primary malignancies (SPMs) can occur in 1.4% to 18% patients, especially when the primary lesion is in the larynx. The most common sites for SPMs are the lungs, the esophagus, and the head and neck region. Treatment of SPMs increases survival. There has been an increased incidence of human papilloma virus (HPV)–associated head and neck cancer in the United States. These HPV-positive tumors are thought to behave differently from non–HPV-positive tumors. HPV-positive patients with head and neck cancer have a significantly better prognosis compared with patients who are HPV negative.

REFERENCES

Argiris A, Karamouzis MV, Raben D, Ferris RL. Head and neck cancer. *Lancet.* 2008;371(9625):1695–1709.

Jones AS, Rafferty M, Fenton JE, et al. Treatment of squamous cell carcinoma of the tongue base: irradiation, surgery, or palliation? *Ann Otol Rhinol Laryngol.* 2007;116(2):92–99.

Kim SY, Roh JL, Yeo NK, et al. Combined 18F-fluorodeoxyglucose-positron emission tomography and computed tomography as a primary screening method for detecting second primary cancers and distant metastases in patients with head and neck cancer. *Ann Oncol.* 2007;18(10):1698–1703.

Snow GB, Annyas AA, van Slooten EA, Bartelink H, Hart AA. Prognostic factors of neck node metastasis. *Clin Otolaryngol Allied Sci.* 1982;7(3):185–192.

Tantiwongkosi B, Yu F, Kanard A, Miller FR. Role of 18F-FDG PET/CT in pre and post treatment evaluation in head and neck carcinoma. *World J Radiol.* 2014;6(5):177.

Case 37

VQ HIGH PROBABILITY

1. d
2. d
3. c
4. a

Discussion

This scan is a high-probability scan for acute pulmonary embolism (PE). There are multiple large, segmental perfusion defects that are mismatched compared with the ventilation images in the right middle lobe and right lower lobe. By PIOPED (Prospective Investigation of Pulmonary Embolism Diagnosis) criteria, there must be at least two large segmental perfusion defects or four moderate segmental perfusion defects that are mismatched in the setting of a clear radiograph. The ventilation images are usually performed before the perfusion images, either with xenon-133 (Xe-133) or Tc-99 DTPA aerosol. Because of the short biologic half-time (T½) in the lungs, Xe-133 imaging can only be performed in one or two projections (two-headed camera), for example, anterior/posterior or, preferably, right and left posterior oblique views, which allow for visualization of three pleural surfaces. This study utilized Xe-133, as can be determined by using a single projection with single-breath, equilibrium, and washout images. The advantage of utilizing Tc-99 DTPA for ventilation is that images can be obtained in all projections, allowing for direct comparison with the perfusion images. Because of the lower ventilation dose retained in the lungs, good Tc-99m macroaggregated albumin (MAA) images can be acquired after the ventilation study. The advantage of Xe-133 is greater sensitivity for detecting obstructive lung disease. A high-probability scan confers a probability of greater than 80% for the presence of acute PE. Low probability signifies a less than 20% probability of PE, and intermediate probability signifies approximately 33%. To determine low or high probability, the chest radiograph should be clear, with no effusion, atelectasis, or infiltrate in the regions of perfusion defects.

A follow-up computed tomographic angiography (CTA) of the chest in this patient demonstrates a central thrombus (filling defect) in the right lower lobe artery.

REFERENCES

Kumar AM, Parker JA. Ventilation/perfusion scintigraphy. *Emerg Med Clin.* 2001;19(4):957–974.

PIOPED Investigators. Value of the ventilation/perfusion scan in acute pulmonary embolism. Results of the prospective investigation of pulmonary embolism diagnosis (PIOPED). *JAMA.* 1990;263(20):2753.

Case 38

THYROID—MULTINODULAR GOITER

1. c
2. d
3. c
4. b

Discussion

This scan has the appearance of multinodular toxic goiter in the clinical context of a hyperthryoid patient, with hot nodules and suppressed non-nodular adjacent thyroid. Nontoxic multinodular goiter would not have suppression of the non-nodular adjacent thyroid. This study may be performed with I-123 or Tc-99m pertechnetate. This is a Tc-99m pertechnetate scan. It appears similar to I-123, but often the Tc-99m pertechnetate scan can be differentiated by visualization of the salivary glands and increased background activity. The degree of radiotracer uptake in the salivary glands is similar to thyroid uptake on Tc-99m pertechnetate scans. The usual administered dose of I-131 for treatment of multinodular goiter is between 20 to 30 mCi, significantly higher than when treating Graves' disease (7–15 mCi). This is because MNG is more resistant to treatment by I-131 than Graves' disease. Once the radiotracer avid nodules are treated (approximately 3–6 months), the remaining gland that was suppressed will function again.

REFERENCE

Ross DS, Burch HB, Cooper DS, et al. 2016 American Thyroid Association guidelines for diagnosis and management of hyperthyroidism and other causes of thyrotoxicosis. *Thyroid.* 2016;26(10):1343–1421.

Case 39

OCTREOSCAN (IN-111 PENTETREOTIDE)—
METASTATIC CARCINOID

1. c
2. c
3. c
4. a

Discussion

This In-111 pentetreotide (OctreoScan) scan shows normal high kidney and renal uptake and intestinal clearance but abnormal uptake in pancreatic neuroendocrine tumors (NETs) and metastases in the liver.

NETs encompass a wide variety of tissue types that produce peptides and hormones causing various clinical symptoms. Well-differentiated NETs express somatostatin receptors (SSTRs) and thus can be imaged with this radiopharmaceutical, which is an eight–amino acid peptide that has high affinity for SSTRs. The overall sensitivity for various NETs varies; carcinoid tumors, gastrinomas, and adrenal medullary tumors have high sensitivity, whereas insulinoma, pituitary adenoma, and meningioma have lower detection sensitivity. False-negative results may occur when the tumors dedifferentiate, resulting in fewer numbers of SSTRs. In those cases, F-18 FDG PET/CT may be of value to identify the tumor.

OctreoScan imaging protocol varies with some institutions acquiring a 4-hour planar images (no bowel activity) in conjunction with delayed 24-hour whole body imaging (bowel clearance). When available, SPECT/CT of the abdomen at 24 hours should be performed for identifying and localizing tumor sites. Tumors that are somatostatin receptor positive may show good response to octreotide (Sandostatin) therapy, but not always.

Ga-68 DOTA-TATE is a newly approved SSTR PET imaging agent. These images are superior to In-111 pentetreotide scans, and the sensitivity for tumor detection is higher. New data have demonstrated encouraging results in treating NETs with lutetium-177 (Lu-177) DOTA-TATE, a beta emitter that binds to SSTRs. Compared with patients on high-dose octreotide therapy, patients with nonresectable NETs receiving this therapy have shown a significant increase in progression-free survival. This is an ideal *theranostic* approach, in which the same somatostatin receptor agent is used, with one radionuclide for diagnosis and another for therapy (Figure 39-1).

REFERENCES

Shi W, Johnston CF, Buchanan KD, et al. Localization of neuroendocrine tumours with [111In] DTPA-octreotide scintigraphy (Octreoscan): a comparative study with CT and MR imaging. *QJM*. 1998;91(4): 295–301.

Strosberg J, El-Haddad G, Wolin KD, et al. Phase 3 Trial of ^{177}Lu-Dotatate for Midgut Neuroendocrine Tumors. *N Engl J Med*. 2017;376(2):125–135. https://doi.org/10.1056/NEJMoa1607427.

Case 40

BONE SCAN—LYTIC LESION

1. b
2. a
3. b
4. a

Discussion

This case demonstrates absent activity in the region of the left sacroiliac joint. This would be defined as a cold defect. When evaluating bone scans for the presence of metastatic disease, it is important to do a systematic search for both hot and cold lesions. Cold (photopenic) lesions are more difficult to detect. Certain cancers are more likely to present with lytic lesions. These include renal cell cancer, thyroid cancer, and multiple myeloma. An isolated photopenic defect on a bone scan is more likely to represent a metastasis compared with an isolated focus of increased radiotracer uptake. In this case, note the absence of the left kidney on the posterior view of the bone scan, indicating prior left nephrectomy for renal cell carcinoma. However, any lytic lesion may be cold on a bone scan. Sometimes, these lesions may not appear hot or cold on a planar bone scan because of their small size and/or overlap of normal bone. SPECT/CT can improve detection.

The photopeak of a radionuclide is not a sharp line but a somewhat broadened peak. This is caused by the imperfect energy resolution of the sodium iodide detector. The window around the photopeak for Tc-99m is usually 15% or 20%, centered around the 140-keV photopeak.

REFERENCE

Parkh JS, Teates CD. Mixed "hot" and "cold" lesions on bone scans. *Semin Nucl Med*. 1992;22(4):289–291.

Case 41

GASTROESOPHAGEAL REFLUX SCINTIGRAPHY

1. b
2. a
3. b
4. d

Discussion

Gastroesophageal reflux is common in the infant population. In most cases, it resolves by age 8 months. However, in a small proportion of the population, reflux may persist with complications, such as strictures, pain, aspiration, and failure to thrive. Other techniques for the diagnosis of reflux, such as endoscopy, the Bernstein acid test, and Tuttle acid reflux test, are used. However, most are invasive and or difficult to perform. The radionuclide study for reflux (milk study) allows for assessment of physiologic activity assessment and quantitation of reflux events, as well as gastric emptying.

This study demonstrates episodic radiotracer migration into the esophagus from the stomach. To perform the test, Tc-99m sulfur colloid is mixed in with the standard formula or breast milk. After ingestion, a rapid frame acquisition of 5 to 10 seconds per frame is performed for 60 minutes. The higher frame rate allows for high sensitivity for detection of reflux disease. The infant should be placed in the supine position, with the camera positioned posteriorly. When performing this study on adults, the radiotracer is mixed with orange juice. To quantify gastric emptying, an initial static image is acquired before starting the rapid acquisition, followed by an image at 60 and 120 minutes. Reflux events can be semiquantified by the number of events, height of reflux into the esophagus, and duration of the event. Alternatively, time–activity curves can be used for detection and quantification. Sensitivity of this study for aspiration is low (<25%). Salivagraphy is considerably more sensitive. It is essentially an esophageal swallow study in which a drop of the radiotracer placed in the posterior pharynx. Normal values for gastric emptying (formula or milk) are approximately 40% to 50% at 1 hour and 60% to 75% at 2 hours.

REFERENCE

Heyman S, Kirkpatrick JA, Winter HS, Treves S. An improved radionuclide method for the diagnosis of gastroesophageal reflux and aspiration in children (milk scan). *Radiology*. 1979;131(2):479–482.

Case 42

RENAL TRANSPLANT—POSTOPERATIVE LEAK

1. c
2. a
3. a
4. b

Discussion

This case demonstrates radiotracer extravasation increasing over time outside the expected regions of radiotracer accumulation (transplanted kidney, ureter, and bladder). This leak extends into the scrotal region. Postoperative urine leak/urinomas are usually diagnosed within the first month after transplantation. The patient may be asymptomatic or present with pain and/or swelling. A fluid collection is a common complication after renal transplantation. Possible etiologies include hematoma, lymphocele, urinoma, or seroma. US is sensitive for the detection of a simple fluid collection but is often unable to identify the etiology of the fluid collection. To diagnose urine leak, renal scintigraphy is ideal. Tc-99m MAG3 is the preferred radiopharmaceutical for the evaluation of renal transplants because of its significant uptake even in the setting of renal dysfunction. It is primarily a renal tubular agent that represents about 80% of renal function. Tc-99m DTPA is dependent on the glomerular filtration rate, which is responsible for only 10% to 20% of renal function. Renal transplants as opposed to native kidneys are imaged in the anterior projection because the renal transplant is in a more anterior location in the pelvis and is closer to the detector in the anterior view. The most likely etiology for this finding in the perioperative period is disruption of the surgical anastomosis. With a slow leak, delayed images may be necessary to document the extravasation.

REFERENCE

Son H, Heiba S, Kostakoglu L, Machac J. Extraperitoneal urine leak after renal transplantation: the role of radionuclide imaging and the value of accompanying SPECT/CT-a case report. *BMC Med Imaging*. 2010;10(1):23.

Case 43

PHEOCHROMOCYTOMA—MIBG

1. a
2. a
3. b
4. b

Discussion

This is an I-123 metaiodobenzylguanidine (MIBG) scan, which demonstrates abnormal increased radiotracer uptake in the region of the right adrenal gland. On the dedicated contrast-enhanced CT scan, this lesion is an extra-adrenal gland, consistent with a paraganglioma.

Pheochromocytomas/paragangliomas can present with symptoms and findings of excessive catecholamines. CT can often localize an adrenal mass and sometimes an extra-adrenal mass. I-123 MIBG can confirm the mass to be a pheochromocytoma or extra-adrenal paraganglioma with high accuracy, and it can detect metastatic disease. Approximately 10% of these tumors occur outside the adrenal gland, with 10% being bilateral and 10% malignant. They can be found anywhere from the bladder up to the base of the skull. They may be associated with multiple endocrine neoplasia syndromes. MIBG has a molecular structure similar to those of norepinephrine and guanethidine. It is taken up in presynaptic adrenergic nerves similar to norepinephrine. Tracer uptake in this tumor is usually quite high. The sensitivity of I-123 MIBG scintigraphy is high (83%–100%), as is the specificity (95%–100%). Numerous drugs can alter the biodistribution of I-123 MIBG, including labetalol and the tricyclic antidepressants nifedipine and reserpine. Hence, a detailed medication history must be performed before scheduling of the patient and, if clinically possible, these drugs withheld. PET/CT imaging with Ga-68 DOTATATE and F18 FDG may better localize disease compared with conventional I-123 MIBG imaging.

REFERENCES

Intenzo CM, Jabbour S, Lin HC, et al. Scintigraphic imaging of body neuroendocrine tumors. *Radiographics*. 2007;27(5):1355–1369.

Janssen I, Blanchet EM, Adams K, et al. Superiority of [68Ga] DOTATATE PET/CT to other functional imaging modalities in the localization of SDHB-associated metastatic pheochromocytoma and paraganglioma. *Clin Cancer Res*. 2015;21(17):3888–3895.

Case 44

F-18 FDG—ATTENUATION CORRECTION

1. b
2. d
3. a
4. b

Discussion

The image shown on the left is the non–attenuation-corrected (NAC) PET image, and the image on the right is the attenuation-corrected (AC) PET image.

During the *emission* portion of the PET scan, detected photons that originate from structures deeper in the body are more highly attenuated by intervening soft tissue compared with those originating closer to the surface. As well, activity originating in the lungs is less attenuated than if surrounded by dense soft tissue. The effects of this attenuation of signal can be seen in the NAC image, where the lungs and skin appear "hot" and activity deeper or more central in the body is relatively lower.

In PET/CT, the *transmission* CT scan is used to construct an attenuation map of density in the body, which can then be used to correct for the absorption of the photons emitted. With dedicated PET-only scanners, the transmission scan is performed with an external positron source (germanium-68 or cesium-137), which rotates around the patient, in a similar fashion as in CT. By comparing the number of photons reaching the PET detectors with and without the patient, an attenuation map can be constructed.

The process of attenuation correction is necessary for SUV determination and for overall image quality. However, artifacts may be introduced by the process of attenuation correction, and thus review of NAC and AC images is sometimes necessary. For example, high-density material (i.e., metal, intravenous [IV] contrast, barium) on CT may falsely cause increased activity on AC PET images. If the activity is not present on NAC images, the apparent increased activity can be attributed to attenuation correction artifact.

Also, respiratory/diaphragmatic motion between the PET scan and the CT scan causes attenuation correction artifacts and anatomic localization artifacts. For example, because of diaphragmatic motion, a liver lesion can erroneously appear at the base of the lung, mimicking a lung nodule. Review of the NAC images may correctly show the location of the lesion.

NAC images are particularly useful for assessing the skin (i.e., melanoma) and peripheral lung nodules which may be more readily detected on NAC images.

REFERENCE

Reinhardt MJ, Wiethoelter N, Matthies A, et al. PET recognition of pulmonary metastases on PET/CT imaging: impact of attenuation-corrected and non-attenuation-corrected PET images. *Eur J Nucl Med Mol Imaging* 2006;33(2):134–139.

Case 45

BONE SCAN SHIN SPLINTS

1. b
2. d
3. a
4. b

Discussion

This case demonstrates a linear focus of increased radiotracer uptake along the posterior medial aspect of the left mid-tibia consistent with shin splints. Shin splints are thought to occur as a result of repetitive trauma/activity resulting in enthesopathy. Patients usually present with complaints of leg soreness related to exercise. Although this case demonstrates unilateral presence of shin splints, in most cases, shin splints are bilateral. On three-phase bone scintigraphy, hyperemia is uncommon in the setting of shin splints, whereas it is common in the setting of a stress fracture. The delayed images in the setting of a stress fracture will demonstrate focal cortical uptake. Bone scintigraphy is very sensitive for the evaluation of frank fractures. Displaced fractures are most commonly diagnosed on radiography or CT. Nondisplaced fractures may be more readily identified on MRI or bone scintigraphy. Most patients undergo MRI evaluations for musculoskeletal trauma. However, in patients who cannot undergo MRI, bone scintigraphy remains a sensitive technique for the evaluation of radiographically occult bone trauma.

REFERENCE

Love C, Din AS, Tomas MB, Kalapparambath TP, Palestro CJ. Radionuclide bone imaging: an illustrative review. *Radiographics*. 2003;23(2):341–358.

Case 46

FDG PET/CT—POOR PREPARATION

1. a
2. a
3. b
4. b

Discussion

This study shows intense diffuse uptake in muscles and the heart and little uptake in the liver. This is consistent with poor preparation. After scanning, patient revealed that he (she) had gone to a fast food restaurant before coming to the PET center. Focal uptake is seen in the right lung, consistent with a lung mass. On repeat scanning (after appropriate preparation [image B]), an additional left femoral lesion could be seen, consistent with osseous metastases.

Standard protocols for F-18 FDG PET/CT recommend a fasting period of 4 to 6 hours before injection. This is because free circulating glucose competes with F-18 FDG for uptake. Fasting reduces serum insulin levels to near-basal levels and thus diminishes FDG uptake by organs such as the heart, muscles, liver, and so on. The serum glucose level should be checked in all patients before imaging, particularly in patients with diabetes. The upper acceptable limits for performing the study should be less than 200-220 mg/dL. False-negative oncologic study results may occur in the setting of elevated serum glucose levels because of decreased uptake of the radiotracer by the tumor. Patients with diabetes must be carefully prepared for the examination. Generally, these patients should not receive long-acting insulin within 12 hours of examination and short-acting insulin within 2 to 4 hours. Although FDG is a glucose analogue, its metabolism is blocked intracellularly. Its primary route of excretion is renal, which is not true of glucose. The optimal imaging time after injection is 45 to 60 minutes. Great care must be taken to standardize imaging delay time so that accurate comparisons can be made between scans on the same patient.

REFERENCE

Cook GJR. Pitfalls in PET/CT interpretation. *Q J Nucl Med Mol Imaging*. 2007;51(3):235.

Case 47

HOT SPOTS

1. c
2. c
3. a
4. d

Discussion

This case demonstrates focal hot spots on Tc-99m MAA perfusion images. This occurs when the technologist or the physician pulls back on a syringe to confirm placement in a vein, thus allowing a small amount of blood to mix with the Tc-99m MAA solution. Tc-99m MAA accelerates blood clotting, causing hot spots to form on the image after injection. It is important to also agitate the syringe just before injections to avoid clumping of MAA, which may also cause hot spots. As well, during injection, it is important to ask the patient to breathe deeply in the supine position to ensure uniform distribution of the radiotracer. If the patient is injected in the upright position, there will be a significant gradient in perfusion as a result of increased flow to the lower lobes.

In a routine VQ study, approximately 200,000 to 400,000 MAA particles are injected into a patient. The MAA particles, on average, range in size from 10 to 30 μm, similar to the precapillary arterioles. These particles obstruct the precapillary arterioles, allowing for imaging approximately 0.1% to 0.3% of vessels. MAA particles degrade over time, with a t½ of 4 to 6 hours. The number of particles may be reduced in certain patients, including neonates, patients with pulmonary hypertension, and pregnant women. Ill effects related to obstruction of precapillary arterioles in the lungs is highly unlikely. Use of a reduced number of particles is advised in patients with right-to-left shunts and pulmonary hypertension, although there have been no reports of ill effects.

REFERENCES

Bajc M, Neilly JB, Miniati M, Schuemichen C, Meignan M, Jonson B. EANM guidelines for ventilation/perfusion scintigraphy. *Eur J Nucl Med Mol Imaging*. 2009;36(8):1356–1370.

Ikehira H, Kinjo M, Yamato Y, et al. Hot spots observed on pulmonary perfusion imaging: a case report. *J Nucl Med Technol*. 1999;27(4): 301–302.

Case 48

PARATHYROID ADENOMA, MEDIASTINAL, TC-99M SESTAMIBI

1. c
2. b
3. d
4. b

Discussion

On the scan, there is normal physiologic uptake in the salivary and lacrimal glands, thyroid, heart, and liver, as well as faint uptake in the nasopharynx. This maximum-intensity projection (MIP) view includes the chest and shows abnormal focal uptake in the mediastinum.

Technetium-99 (Tc-99m) sestamibi, Tc-99m Pertechnetate and indium-123 (I-123) metaiodobenzylguanidine (MIBG) may show thyroid uptake. In-111 WBC scan does not demonstrate physiologic uptake in the thyroid gland. Myocardial wall uptake makes this a Tc-99m Sestamibi scan.

Tc-99m sestamibi study can be used to localize an autonomous hyperfunctioning parathyroid adenoma in patients with primary hyperparathyroidism presenting with serum hypercalcemia and hypophosphatemia. The radiotracer localizes and is retained in mitochondria. Uptake of Tc-99m sestamibi is postulated to be based on the high number of mitochondria in the oxyphil cells of an adenoma. Normal functioning parathyroid glands are not usually seen on imaging.

Tc-99m sestamibi is particularly useful in the detection of ectopic tissue in the mediastinum and in the upper neck. This is a case of mediastinal parathyroid adenoma seen as focal radiotracer uptake in the chest. Tc-99m sestamibi scans are important to perform for preoperative planning. Asymmetric appearance of the thyroid gland was related to asymmetry in relative thyroid gland size, that is, the right lobe being larger than the left lobe.

REFERENCES

Lavely WC, Goetze S, Friedman KP, et al. Comparison of SPECT/CT, SPECT, and planar parathyroid imaging with single- and dual-phase Tc-99m sestamibi parathyroid scintigraphy. *J Nucl Med.* 2007;48(7):1084–1089.

Rubello D, Casara D, Fiore D, Muzzio P, Zonzin G, Shapiro B. An ectopic mediastinal parathyroid adenoma accurately located by a single-day imaging protocol of Tc-99m pertechnetate–MIBI subtraction scintigraphy and MIBI-SPECT–computed tomographic image fusion. *Clin Nucl Med.* 2002;27(3):186–190.

Case 49

BONE SCAN AFTER MUGA

1. b
2. b
3. d
4. d

Discussion

The scan demonstrates symmetric uptake throughout the skeletal system, with activity in the renal collecting systems and urinary bladder. The anterior view as well shows surface contamination of the external genitalia—all findings consistent with a bone scan performed with Tc-99m–labeled diphosphonate.

There is additional, unexpected extraosseous activity in the heart, vessels, liver, and spleen. Extraosseous activity may occur for a variety of reasons. In this case, the clinical history is particularly important. A multigated acquisition (MUGA) scan performed earlier in the day would account for all the areas of extraosseous activity. A MUGA study is most commonly used to determine left ventricular ejection fraction (LVEF) in patients receiving cardiotoxic drugs, such as doxorubicin. Gated blood pool ventriculography utilizes Tc-99m–labeled RBCs, which distributes to the heart, vessels, liver, and spleen. One would expect to see bowel activity after a Tc-99m Sestamibi study and no cardiac activity on an In-111 WBC study making these choices less likely.

Extraosseous soft tissue activity may occur from impurities in Tc-labeled diphosphonate compounds. Free Tc-99m pertechnetate accounts for activity in the thyroid, stomach, and oropharynx. Colloid impurities may result in liver activity.

Other common causes of extraosseous soft tissue activity may result from other pathologic conditions. Diphosphonates bind to calcium phosphate salts, which can form from calcium and phosphate that leak into the extracellular fluid from hypoxic or dead cells. This process may account for uptake of the tracer in metastatic disease where there is cell necrosis or areas of infarction.

REFERENCES

Love C, Din AS, Tomas MB, Kalapparambath TP, Palestro CJ. Radionuclide bone imaging: an illustrative review. *Radiographics.* 2003;23(2):341–358.
Virmani S, Virmani R, Singh J, Ali A. Osseous and extra-osseous uptake patterns on a bone scan: a pictorial review. *J Nucl Med.* 2015;56 (suppl 3):1927.

Case 50

THYROIDITIS, CHRONIC LYMPHOCYTIC THYROIDITIS, F-18 FDG PET

1. d
2. b
3. a
4. c

Discussion

There is diffuse uptake in the thyroid gland on this positron-emission tomography (PET) scan. In this patient with no known history of thyroid disease, statistically, the most likely diagnosis is chronic lymphocytic thyroiditis (Hashimoto's thyroiditis). Normally, there is no uptake of FDG in the thyroid gland. Graves' disease and subacute thyroiditis could look similar.

Incidental, diffuse uptake in the thyroid gland on FDG PET scan has been reported in 0.6% to 3.3% of patients undergoing FDG PET or PET/CT and commonly represents benign disease. In one large retrospective study, out of 4732 investigated FDG-PET/CT scans, 138 (2.9%) had diffuse thyroid uptake, and greater than 50% of these patients had chronic lymphocytic thyroiditis with or without hypothyroidism.

Chronic lymphocytic thyroiditis is characterized by diffuse infiltration of stroma between follicles with lymphocytes and plasma cells. Diagnosis can be made by detection of specific antibodies, antithyroid peroxidase, and antithyroglobulin. Clinically, patients are often euthyroid with normal T_3 and T_4 hormones. Some may be hypothyroid. Hashimoto's thyroiditis is more common in women (F/M = 9:1). Thyroid gland may be enlarged and, as shown by ultrasonography (US), heterogeneous in echogenicity with increased vascularity. Nodules may also be present. In later stages, the gland may become small, heterogeneous, and echogenic with associated clinical hypothyroidism.

Patients may be treated with levothyroxin in the setting of hypothyroidism. Although rare, there is an increased risk of developing thyroid non-Hodgkin's lymphoma (NHL). Among patients with Hashimoto's thyroiditis, the risk of thyroid lymphoma is at least 60 times higher than in patients without thyroiditis.

REFERENCES

Karantanis D, Bogsrud TV, Wiseman GA, et al. Clinical significance of diffusely increased 18F-FDG uptake in the thyroid gland. *J Nucl Med.* 2007;48(6):896–901.

Kurata S, Ishibashi M, Hiromatsu Y, et al. Diffuse and diffuse-plus-focal uptake in the thyroid gland identified by using FDG-PET: prevalence of thyroid cancer and Hashimoto's thyroiditis. *Ann Nucl Med.* 2007;21(6):325–330.

Case 51

LUNG PERFUSION SCAN—RIGHT-TO-LEFT SHUNT

1. b
2. c
3. d
4. b

Discussion

This examination was performed to evaluate for underlying right-to-left shunt in a patient with atrial septal defect. To perform this scan, a patient is injected with Tc-99m macroaggregated albumin (MAA) through peripheral intravenous (IV) administration. Particle size ranges from 10 to 90 μm, with a mean of 30 to 40 μm. The particles occlude arteriolar capillary beds, allowing for imaging. Less than 0.1% capillary beds are occluded, so the patients are not symptomatic, and no ill effects can occur. In addition, the dual circulation of the lungs prevents pulmonary infarction.

Brain activity should not be seen on a normal scan and is diagnostic of a right-to-left shunt. Increased uptake in the kidneys may also be caused by the presence of a shunt. Visualization of the thyroid (not seen here) and kidneys in the same scan may result from the presence of free pertechnetate, most likely related to breakdown of the radiopharmaceutical. It is best to inject a freshly prepared radiopharmaceutical. The percentage of shunting can be calculated. Common causes for shunting include congenital heart defects, such as atrial septal defect and ventricular septal defects, or hepatopulmonary syndrome. Some institution may reduce the number of particles injected if a large shunt is possible.

REFERENCES

Barasch M, Rickley C, Intenzo C, Kim S. Imaging approach in patients with right to left shunting. *J Nucl Med*. 2017;58(suppl 1):1138.

Marashdeh W, Wahl RL. Case report: brown fat accumulation of Tc-99m macroaggregated albumin in a lung perfusion study in a patient with multiple lung arteriovenous malformations and right-to-left shunting. *Medicine*. 2015;94(42):e1820.

Case 52

PITUITARY ADENOMA—F-18 FDG PET/CT

1. b
2. d
3. a
4. b

Discussion

The F-18 FDG PET/CT images show focal increased activity in the right aspect of the sella turcica, the site of the pituitary gland. On the CT images, no discrete mass is seen. Of note, the MIP image shows no other abnormal uptake in the remainder of the body. The coronal postcontrast magnetic resonance imaging (MRI) scan demonstrates a rounded hypo-enhancing nodule (approximately 10 mm), relative to the remainder of the pituitary gland, in the right aspect of the pituitary gland, consistent with a pituitary microadenoma.

Retrospective studies have reported a wide range for the incidence of incidental pituitary uptake on FDG PET/CT scans, between 0.07% and 0.8%. Differences in incidence are likely secondary to varying technique, misregistration in the head/neck region, and interobserver variability. The normal pituitary gland does not demonstrate significant increased FDG uptake. As the scanner technology improves, mild uniform uptake may be seen in the pituitary gland.

In previous studies and case reports, among those with focal pituitary uptake, pituitary adenoma (either microadenomas or macroadenomas) was the most common pathologic etiology, with rare instances of metastatic disease or inflammatory uptake. A few of the studies have suggested a cutoff maximum standardized uptake value (SUV_{max}) of 4 as a guideline in differentiating pathologic uptake from nonspecific, physiologic uptake.

In patients with a primary malignancy and disseminated metastatic disease, focal uptake may, in fact, be caused by a pituitary metastasis. In rare cases, differentiation between a solitary metastatic lesion and an adenoma may not possible via imaging alone. Other rare inflammatory conditions of the pituitary, such as lymphocytic hypophysitis and Langerhans' cell histiocytosis—diagnoses made clinically or by pathologic examination, rather than by imaging—may also cause uptake.

Ultimately, focal, increased FDG activity in the region of the pituitary on PET/CT scans warrants further diagnostic evaluation with MRI and clinical evaluation.

REFERENCES

Hyun SH, Choi JY, Lee KH, Choe YS, Kim BT. Incidental focal 18F-FDG uptake in the pituitary gland: clinical significance and differential diagnostic criteria. *J Nucl Med.* 2011;52(4):547–550.

Jeong SY, Lee SW, Lee HJ, et al. Incidental pituitary uptake on whole-body 18F-FDG PET/CT: a multicentre study. *Eur J Nucl Med Mol Imaging.* 2010;37(12):2334–2343.

Case 53

LYMPHOSCINTIGRAPHY—LYMPHATIC OBSTRUCTION

1. b
2. a
3. d
4. b

Discussion

After injection of Tc-99m sulfur colloid (SC) into the interdigital web spaces of both feet, whole-body anterior and posterior scintigraphy at 4 hours demonstrates delayed and diminished flow in the right leg. No lymphatic trunk or collaterals are seen in the right leg. There is absence of uptake in expected location of right ilioinguinal lymph nodes compared with uptake on the left side. On the delayed 4-hour images, there is dermal backflow in the right foot and ankle. Findings are consistent with lymphatic obstruction of the right lower extremity.

Lymphedema is the abnormal accumulation of lymphatic fluid in the interstitial spaces of the skin resulting in soft tissue edema as a result of obstructed transport of lymph through the lymphatic system. Symptoms include extremity swelling, decreased mobility, and secondary infections. The disorder typically affects the dermis and spares the deeper compartments.

Lymphedema may be primary or secondary. Primary causes include congenital or genetic causes resulting in pathologic development of lymphatic vessels. Secondary causes include prior lymphadenectomy, radiation, postinfectious (i.e., filariasis), compression of lymphatics by tumor, or tumor infiltration into the lymphatic system. The differential diagnosis of suspected extremity lymphedema includes obesity, venous disease, and systemic disease (e.g., hypoalbuminemia).

Lymphoscintigraphy is the primary imaging modality used in determining a diagnosis in patients with suspected extremity lymphedema. For the lower extremities, filtered Tc-99m SC is injected into the interdigital web spaces of the patient's feet, creating a wheal. To aid in lymphatic return, patient may walk or the injection region massaged. Sweep of the chest, abdomen, pelvis, and bilateral lower extremities in anterior and posterior projections is performed. Delayed images are obtained as clinically necessary.

Normal scintigraphic findings include symmetric, bilateral lymphatic uptake of radiotracer and visualization of the ilioinguinal nodes. Lymphedema findings include delayed uptake of radiotracer in the extremity of interest despite exercise, dermal backflow (stocking sign) in the extremity, presence of collateral and/or dilated lymphatic channels, interruption of lymphatic channels, and absent or asymmetric visualization of lymph nodes and lymphatic trunks.

REFERENCES

Hassanein AH, Maclellan RA, Grant FD, Greene AK. Diagnostic accuracy of lymphoscintigraphy for lymphedema and analysis of false-negative tests. *Plast Reconstr Surg Glob Open*. 2017;5(7):e1396.

Moshiri M, Katz DS, Boris M, Yung E. Using lymphoscintigraphy to evaluate suspected lymphedema of the extremities. *Am J Roentgenol*. 2002;178(2):405–412.

Case 54

GI BLEED

1. b
2. d
3. b
4. d

Discussion

Dynamic 1-minute images from the case above demonstrate new activity (row 1, image 4) arising in the left abdomen, which increases over time, conforms to the lumen and distribution of the small bowel (likely the jejunum, given the location), and appears to move antegrade and retrograde—all of which are criteria for diagnosis of bleeding site for Tc-99m RBC scintigraphy.

There are several pitfalls that may cause misinterpretations and false-positive studies. Importantly, a region of fixed activity should not be interpreted as active bleeding.

Fixed activity may be caused by regions of physiologic uptake in the genitourinary system, with physiologic activity in the renal collecting system or urinary bladder. As well, uptake in the uterus may occur during menses, and penile blood pool may be misinterpreted as rectal bleeding. A lateral view is useful in differentiating the location of midline pelvic activity.

Vascular structures (i.e., varices, grafts, aneurysms), splenosis, or regions of inflammation may also demonstrate fixed activity. Free pertechnetate resulting from poor labeling may also cause gastric uptake that moves into the small and large bowels, mimicking a gastric hemorrhage. Imaging of the salivary and thyroid glands can confirm or exclude free pertechnetate as the cause of the gastric uptake.

Various methods can be used to label RBCs, allowing Tc-99m to bind to the beta chain of the hemoglobin molecule. However, if these methods are not available, scintigraphy for GI bleeding can also be performed by using Tc-99m SC, which is rapidly cleared from the intravascular space by the reticuloendothelial system. The circulating half-life in patients with normal liver function is between 2 to 3 minutes, and by 15 to 20 minutes there is effectively no Tc-99m left in the blood pool, allowing clear visualization of extravasated isotope at the bleeding site. Major disadvantage of this method, however, is that bleeding must be active at the time of injection.

With both tracer methods, bleeding rates of approximately 0.05 to 0.1 mL/min have been detected. Conventional angiography has been reported to detect bleeding rates of 1.0 mL/min or greater.

REFERENCES

Grady E. Gastrointestinal bleeding scintigraphy in the early 21st century. *J Nucl Med.* 2016;57(2):252–259.

Howarth DM. The role of nuclear medicine in the detection of acute gastrointestinal bleeding. *Semin Nucl Med.* 2006;36(2):133–146.

Case 55

F-18 FDG PET SCAN—VOCAL CORD PARALYSIS

1. c
2. a
3. c
4. b

Discussion

Vocal cord paralysis caused by recurrent laryngeal nerve dysfunction can be a sign of mediastinal disease and, in a patient with a prior history of malignancy, an indication of tumor recurrence.

The CT image at the level of the vocal cords shows medialization of the left posterior vocal cord margin and air distending the left laryngeal ventricle caused by thyroarytenoid muscle atrophy. As a result, the airway has the shape similar to a ship's sail ("sail sign"). These CT findings are consistent with left vocal cord paralysis. The PET/CT fused image shows asymmetric activity in the normal right cord resulting from compensatory hypertrophy of the nonparalyzed muscles.

In this patient with a prior history of left upper lobectomy for malignancy, there is also focal uptake at the anastomosis with hypermetabolic soft tissue infiltration into the adjacent mediastinum at the aorticopulmonary window, the site of the where the left recurrent laryngeal nerve courses.

REFERENCES

Lee M, Lilien DL, Ramaswamy MR, Nathan CAO. Unilateral vocal cord paralysis causes contralateral false-positive positron emission tomography scans of the larynx. *Ann Otol Rhinol Laryngol.* 2005;114(3):202–206.

Paquette CM, Manos DC, Psooy BJ. Unilateral vocal cord paralysis: a review of CT findings, mediastinal causes, and the course of the recurrent laryngeal nerves. *Radiographics.* 2012;32(3):721–740.

Case 56

F-18 FDG PET SCAN—ENDOMETRIAL CANCER

1. d
2. b
3. d
4. d

Discussion

Endometrial cancer is the most commonly diagnosed gynecologic malignancy in the developed countries, with a peak incidence between ages 55 and 65 years. Risk factors for endometrial cancer are those that increase a woman's exposure to unopposed estrogen over her lifetime. Thus, common risk factors include obesity, nulliparity, anovulatory cycles, and tamoxifen.

Most patients diagnosed with endometrial cancer have early-stage disease confined to the uterus and do not require imaging. MRI, CT, or PET/CT is indicated in those with more advanced disease and those who have the more aggressive histologic subtypes (grade 3 endometrioid, serous and clear cell) and are at higher risk for metastatic adenopathy.

Compared with MRI, PET/CT has a limited role for local staging of primary cancer, whereas PET/CT is a useful technique for assessing distant metastases throughout the whole body in a single examination in patients with advanced-stage disease and for detection of recurrent disease.

In this patient with an aggressive endometrioid tumor and a biopsy-proven metastatic inguinal lymph node, the stage is consistent with stage IV because the metastatic inguinal nodes are regarded as M1 disease.

REFERENCES

Alonso O, Taroco MR, Damian A, Castro R, Engler H. Role of 18F-FDG PET/CT for the detection of recurrent disease in patients with endometrial adenocarcinoma. *J Nucl Med*. 2017;58(suppl 1):354.

Kitajima K, Murakami K, Kaji Y, Sugimura K. Spectrum of FDG PET/CT findings of uterine tumors. *Am J Roentgenol*. 2010;195(3):737–743.

Case 57

RENAL SCAN—DMSA SCARRING

1. b
2. c
3. a
4. b

Discussion

Tc-99m dimercaptosuccinic acid (DMSA) is used to image the renal parenchyma and typically utilized to evaluate for cortical scarring/pyelonephritis and to demonstrate differential renal function.

DMSA binds to the sulfhydryl groups in proximal tubules at the renal cortex, rather than agents that are either filtered at the glomerulus (diethylenetriaminepentaacetic acid [DTPA]), or secreted by the proximal tubules (mercaptoacetyltriglycine [MAG3]). Background clearance is slow, and the kidney clears a small percentage of the tracer, allowing delayed static images of the kidney to be acquired. Pinhole collimator imaging allows for high-resolution imaging of the renal cortex.

In the images shown, the posterior planar view demonstrates asymmetric decreased activity in the right renal parenchyma. The magnified image of the right kidney demonstrates multiple cortical defects. These findings could be seen with acute pyelonephritis, but if persistent over months, it is more consistent with scarring.

Scarring is associated with vesicoureteral reflux and infection. It is caused by the failure of the vesicoureteral valve. Reflux may resolve spontaneously as the child grows. Renal damage and scarring is more likely to occur in patients with severe reflux disease. Underlying infection is a prerequisite for renal damage because sterile urine will not cause renal injury. Siblings of patients with reflux disease are at increased risk of also having reflux disease.

REFERENCES

Mattoo TK, Chesney RW, Greenfield SP, et al. Renal scarring in the randomized intervention for children with vesicoureteral reflux (RIVUR) trial. *Clin J Am Soc Nephrol*. 2016;11(1):54–61. 2015.

Rushton HG, Majd MASSOUD, Jantausch B, Wiedermann BL, Belman AB. Renal scarring following reflux and nonreflux pyelonephritis in children: evaluation with 99mtechnetium-dimercaptosuccinic acid scintigraphy. *J Urol*. 1992;147(5):1327–1332.

Case 58

INDIUM 111 DTPA—NORMAL PRESSURE HYDROCEPHALUS (NPH)

1. c
2. d
3. d
4. b

Discussion

In radionuclide cisternography, the radiopharmaceutical, Indium-111 (In-111) DTPA is injected intrathecally into the lumbar subarachnoid space via lumbar puncture, and multiple planar images are taken over a period of hours to days to track the flow of cerebrospinal fluid (CSF).

CSF is predominantly secreted by the choroid plexuses of the lateral, third, and fourth ventricles. After leaving the fourth ventricle, CSF flows around the brainstem, cerebellum, and hemispheres and back up to the basal cisterns. CSF is then absorbed through the arachnoid villi, which drain into the parasagittal venous sinuses.

In-111 DTPA is an ideal tracer to track CSF flow because it is not lipid soluble and not absorbed across the ependyma before reaching the arachnoid villi, where it is cleared. The half-life of 67 hours allows for prolonged imaging.

In a normal patient, after injection, the tracer reaches the basal cisterns by 1 hour, the frontal poles and Sylvian fissures by 2 to 6 hours, the cerebral convexities by 12 hours, and the arachnoid villi in the sagittal sinus by 24 hours. Normally, the tracer should not enter the ventricles because physiologic flow is in the opposite direction. This case demonstrates tracer activity within the ventricular system, with no to minimal radiotracer flow over the convexities; this is consistent with the diagnosis of communication hydrocephalus, or normal pressure hydrocephalus (NPH).

NPH is a form of communicating hydrocephalus. The classic clinical triad includes progressive dementia, ataxia, and urinary incontinence. Usually, these findings, normal CSF pressures, and radiographic evidence of ventriculomegaly are required to make the diagnosis

In patients with normal pressure hydrocephalus, there is impairment of the reabsorption of the CSF by the arachnoid granulations and reversal of CSF flow. The classic findings of NPH include abnormal reflux of radiotracer into the ventricles and absence of activity over the convexities on delayed images. The ventricular reflux persists for 24 to 48 hours or more, with little or no flow of the tracer over the convexities. It has been suggested that patients with this pattern of uptake may benefit from surgical shunting. However, not all patients improve after the procedure.

REFERENCES

Gallia GL, Rigamonti D, Williams MA. The diagnosis and treatment of idiopathic normal pressure hydrocephalus. *Nat Clin Pract Neurol.* 2006;2(7):375–381.

Thut DP, Kreychman A, Obando JA. 111In-DTPA cisternography with SPECT/CT for the evaluation of normal pressure hydrocephalus. *J Nucl Med Technol.* 2014;42(1):70–74.

Case 59

HEPATOPULMONARY SHUNT— RADIOEMBOLIZATION PLANNING

1. b
2. c
3. c
4. c

Discussion

Catheter-directed, arterial delivery of radioactive Yttrium-90 (Y-90)–labeled microspheres has been used to treat hepatocellular carcinoma and metastatic liver disease because these neoplasms are primarily supplied by the hepatic artery. The microspheres are, on average, 20 to 40 microns in diameter and become lodged in the peritumoral and intratumoral arterial vasculature. Y-90 emits pure high-energy beta rays with an average penetration range of 2.5 mm and a maximum range of 11 mm in tissue and thus allows for local delivery of radiation to the tumor while minimizing exposure to the normal liver parenchyma. Y-90–microsphere therapy is approved by the U.S. Food and Drug Administration (FDA) for the treatment of unresectable hepatocellular carcinoma and metastatic colorectal cancer.

Two absolute contraindications to microsphere-based Y-90 treatment are exaggerated hepatopulmonary shunting (usually >20%) and reflux into the arteries that supply the gastroduodenal region. If the shunt fraction is 10%, the dose to be administered may be reduced. Hepatopulmonary shunting may occur as a result of abnormal liver tumor vasculature with arteriovenous shunting. If this shunting is significant, treatment with Y-90 microspheres may cause pulmonary insufficiency resulting from radiation pneumonitis. Additionally, reflux of the microspheres into the vascular supply of the gastrointestinal (GI) tract may lead to ulceration and ischemic complications.

These conditions may be detected at scintigraphy with the injection of 5 to 6 mCi of Tc-99m–labeled MAA as a microsphere surrogate into the hepatic arterial territory.

The hepatopulmonary shunt fraction is calculated as a percentage of the counts in the lung over the total counts in the lung and liver. Patients in whom the hepatopulmonary shunt fraction is greater than 20% of the injected dose or in whom the shunt fraction indicates potential exposure of the lung to an absorbed radiation dose of more than 30 Gy are not considered for treatment with Y-90 microspheres. Additional exclusion criteria include blood flow toward the GI region that is not correctable by embolization or catheter positioning.

In this case, planar scintigram obtained after hepatic arterial injection of 5 mCi (185 MBq) of Tc-99m–labeled MAA showed radionuclide activity in regions of interest in the liver and lungs but not in the GI region.

REFERENCE

Gulec SA, Mesoloras G, Dezarn WA, McNeillie P, Kennedy AS. Safety and efficacy of Y-90 microsphere treatment in patients with primary and metastatic liver cancer: the tumor selectivity of the treatment as a function of tumor to liver flow ratio. *J Transl Med.* 2007;5(1):15.

Case 60

F-18 FDG PET—LARGE VESSEL VASCULITIS

1. a
2. c
3. d
4. c

Discussion

The sagittal view of the FDG PET scan shows intense, homogeneous uptake in the wall of the ascending and descending thoracic aorta and the abdominal aorta, as well as in the visualized great vessels. Given the patient's clinical history and symptoms, findings are consistent with giant cell arteritis, a large vessel vasculitis (LVV). The uniform diffuse uptake in the vasculature makes vasculitis the most likely diagnosis.

LVV involves inflammation of aorta and major branch vessels. The pathologic hallmark of LVV is the presence of chronic inflammatory lesions within the vessel wall. FDG accumulates in the inflammatory cells as a result of overexpression of glucose transporters (GLUTs) and activation of glycolytic enzymes. On FDG PET, LVV is depicted by homogeneously increased activity in walls of large arteries (aorta, iliac, femoral, subclavian, carotid). Atherosclerotic disease, however, may show no activity or mild heterogeneous activity with skipped regions.

Two syndromes account for most cases of LVV: giant cell arteritis (GCA) and Takayasu's arteritis.

Studies suggest that FDG PET may diagnose vasculitis when other diagnostic tests are equivocal or negative. For example, in patients with suspected giant cell arteritis, but with a negative temporal artery biopsy, FDG PET may show large vessel involvement indicative of GCA. As well, FDG PET aids in depicting extent of disease and may be useful for monitoring response to therapy.

The limited resolution of PET/CT (4 mm) limits detection of small- and medium-vessel vasculitides, such as polyarteritis nodosa.

REFERENCES

James OG, Christensen JD, Wong TZ, Borges-Neto S, Koweek LM. Utility of FDG PET/CT in inflammatory cardiovascular disease. *Radiographics.* 2011;31(5):1271–1286.

Zerizer I, Tan K, Khan S, et al. Role of FDG-PET and PET/CT in the diagnosis and management of vasculitis. *Eur J Radiol.* 2010;73(3):504–509.

Case 61

LIPOMATOUS HYPERTROPHY OF THE INTERATRIAL SEPTUM

1. d
2. a
3. d
4. b

Discussion

The PET/CT images demonstrate activity between the right and left atria in the interatrial septum, which, on the CT image, is thickened and of fat attenuation on CT. This is known as *lipomatous hypertrophy of the interatrial septum* (LHIS).

Differential considerations of fat-containing lesions in the heart include lipoma, liposarcoma, and arrhythmogenic right ventricular dysplasia (ARVD). Myxoma is the most common primary cardiac neoplasm but does not have features of fat on CT, is usually connected to the septum by a stalk, and is mobile.

LHIS is not a neoplasm, but deposition of increased amounts of fat in the interatrial septum. LHIS has been described having a characteristic dumbbell-shaped lesion sparing the fossa ovalis.

LHIS is an uncommon entity, often discovered incidentally on imaging in asymptomatic individuals. However, LHIS may present as obstructive right atrial mass and exertional dyspnea, and there is a rare association with LHIS with supraventricular arrhythmia and sudden death. Prevalence increases with age and is associated with obesity.

It has been postulated that the moderate increased activity, sometimes seen on PET images, may be caused by variable amounts of brown fat in the lesion. However, there are alternative theories to the etiology of the activity, including possible inflammation. Nonetheless, knowledge of this entity is important to avoid misdiagnosis of a malignant lesion.

REFERENCES

Fan CM, Fischman AJ, Kwek BH, et al. Lipomatous hypertrophy of the interatrial septum: increased uptake on FDG PET. *AJR Am J Roentgenol.* 2005;184(1):339–342.

Zukotynski KA, Israel DA, Kim CK. FDG uptake in lipomatous hypertrophy of the interatrial septum is not likely related to brown adipose tissue. *Clin Nucl Med.* 2011;36(9):767–769.

Case 62

INDIUM WBC—VERTEBRAL OSTEOMYELITIS

1. c
2. d
3. d
4. c

Discussion

Leukocytes, or white blood cells (WBCs), are the primary cellular components in the response to infection and inflammation. Leukocytes include granulocytes (neutrophils, basophils, and eosinophils), monocytes, and lymphocytes. With in vitro labeling with In-111 oxine, all components are labeled, although the majority of cells labeled are neutrophils. The final preparation also contains 10% to 20% labeled platelets and erythrocytes.

Routine imaging for infection is typically performed at 24 hours. At this time, the highest uptake is in the spleen, followed by the liver and bone marrow. For detection of inflammatory bowel disease, imaging is performed earlier at 4 hours, because the inflamed mucosal cells are shed into the bowel and the location of the inflammation at the time of imaging may be erroneous.

Typically, an area of infection/inflammation on an In-111 WBC study presents as activity outside the normal distribution or as an area of increased relative uptake. However, in cases of vertebral osteomyelitis, the In-111 WBC study has a high false-negative rate. Normal or decreased uptake may be seen at the site of infection, as seen in this case. Absence of uptake may be secondary to slow blood flow in a region of thrombosis, pus, or infarction. Because there is a high false-negative rate (40%) with In-111 leukocytes, gallium-67 (Ga-67), or fluorine-18 (F-18), FDG PET/CT should be used for the evaluation of spinal infections.

REFERENCES

Palestro CJ. Radionuclide imaging of osteomyelitis. *Semin Nucl Med*. WB Saunders. 2015;45(1):32–46.

Palestro CJ. Radionuclide imaging of musculoskeletal infection: a review. *J Nucl Med*. 2016;57(9):1406–1412.

Case 63

THYROID SCAN—LINGUAL THYROID

1. a
2. b
3. c
4. d

Discussion

Frontal and lateral planar images from a Tc-99m pertechnetate scan of the patient's head, neck, and upper chest are shown. There is focal nodular accumulation of tracer at the base of the tongue and absence of focal uptake in the expected region of the normal thyroid in the neck. Findings are consistent with ectopic thyroid tissue—a lingual thyroid.

Lingual thyroid tissue is an uncommon embryologic anomaly, which results from failure of the thyroid anlage, during the first trimester, to descend from the foramen cecum at the base of the tongue to its normal prelaryngeal site. The thyroid anlage normally descends in the midline of the neck, first coursing anteriorly to the primordial hyoid bone and then looping inferiorly and posteriorly to the hyoid bone before continuing its descent into the infrahyoid portion of the neck, anterior to the thyrohyoid membrane, thyroid cartilage, and trachea. Theoretically, ectopic thyroid tissue may be found anywhere along this course.

The base of the tongue is the most common location for ectopic thyroid tissue, accounting for roughly 90% of reported cases. In approximately 75% of patients with a lingual thyroid, this ectopic tissue is the only functioning thyroid tissue. Thus, imaging of the lower neck and upper thorax is necessary to look for a normal thyroid gland.

Patients with lingual thyroid tissue are often asymptomatic but may present with a neck mass, dysphagia, obstructive sleep apnea, or dysphonia. Patients may be euthyroid or hypothyroid. There is a gender predilection—four times more common in females. The ectopic tissue may enlarge rapidly during puberty.

Imaging for evaluation of ectopic thyroid tissue can be performed with either Tc-99m pertechnetate or I-123. In children, Tc-99m pertechnetate is preferred because of ease of protocol (20 minute imaging after IV injection) and decreased radiation dose compared with I-123. I-123 can be administered orally but requires a 4- to 6-hour uptake period before imaging. Frontal and lateral views, including the head/neck and the base of tongue, as well as the lower neck/upper chest to image the normal area of the thyroid, should be obtained.

Therapy with levothyroxine and surgical excision are mainstays of symptomatic lingual thyroid therapy, but radioiodine therapy is also effective in relieving symptoms and is preferred in select cases.

REFERENCES

Gandhi A, Wong KK, Gross M, Avram A. Successful ablation of lingual thyroid imaged with SPECT/CT and treated with radioactive iodine-131 avoiding surgery and its associated risks. *J Nucl Med.* 2015;56(suppl 3):1644.

Zander DA, Smoker WR. Imaging of ectopic thyroid tissue and thyroglossal duct cysts. *Radiographics.* 2014;34(1):37–50.

Case 64

BONE SCAN—LIVER METASTASES

1. d
2. b
3. b
4. c

Discussion

In this case, the whole body bone scan shows focal uptake in the right upper quadrant of the abdomen in the expected region of the liver. A second focus is also evident on the anterior view only in the midline abdomen, indicating that the uptake is located more anteriorly, thus excluding the possibility of a lesion in the spine. Both foci were found to correspond to metastatic liver lesions from a colonic neoplasm seen on dedicated CT (not pictured).

Liver uptake on a bone scan may result from variety of reasons. If there is a history of malignancy, heterogeneous uptake in the liver is more suggestive of primary and metastatic disease. Other pathophysiologic conditions, such as amyloidosis or hepatic necrosis, have been reported as showing diffuse hepatic uptake on the bone scan.

A recent nuclear medicine scan (i.e., Tc-99m SC or Tc-99m–labeled WBC) may account for diffuse uptake in the liver, although one would expect to also see uptake in the spleen.

Faulty preparation of the radiopharmaceutical may also be a cause. Excess alumina from the technetium generator eluate may lead to colloid formation, which can accumulate in the reticulo-endothelial system and present as diffuse uptake in the liver.

Many factors affect the localization of Tc-99m methyl diphosphonate (MDP) in the extraosseous soft tissues. After IV injection, radiopharmaceutical localization is dependent on regional blood flow and vascularity, as well as the extracellular fluid compartment into which the tracer quickly distributes. Once within the soft tissues, the Tc-99m MDP concentration in tissues is known to be related to the formation of calcium phosphate salts from calcium and phosphate that leak into the extracellular fluid from hypoxic or dead cells. These salts bind to the diphosphonates. This process may account for the uptake in pathophysiologic disease states of the liver. It was also noted, incidentally, on this scan that there was delayed excretion of radiotracer in the left kidney corresponding to mild hydronephrosis seen on a subsequent renal ultrasound image (not pictured).

REFERENCES

Cai L, Chen Y, Huang Z, Wu J. Incidental detection of solitary hepatic metastasis by 99mTc-MDP and 18F-NaF PET/CT in a patient with osteosarcoma of the tibia. *Clin Nucl Med*. 2015;40(9):759–761.

Loutfi I, Collier BD, Mohammed AM. Nonosseous abnormalities on bone scans. *J Nucl Med Technol*. 2003;31(3):149–153.

Case 65

F-18 FDG PET SCAN—THYMIC REBOUND

1. c
2. a
3. d
4. a

Discussion

On the axial fused FDG PET/CT images, there is diffuse uptake in the anterior mediastinum corresponding to triangular-shaped soft tissue that conforms to the shape of the anterior mediastinum. Given the history of fairly recent chemotherapy and no other FDG-avid lesions in the body, findings reflect thymic rebound hyperplasia. FDG avidity may be seen in normal thymus in younger patient populations, usually 20 years and younger.

After the body is exposed to stress (i.e., chemotherapy, radiation), the thymus may atrophy, to as little as 40% of its original volume. During recovery, the thymus may return to its original size and can grow to be as much as 50% larger—a phenomenon known as *thymic rebound hyperplasia*. Among patients who receive chemotherapy, roughly 10% to 25% may develop rebound hyperplasia, usually occurring within 2 years of initiation of chemotherapy.

Distinguishing thymic hyperplasia from recurrent or metastatic tumors is dependent on the morphology of the lesion on the CT image.

Thymic rebound hyperplasia typically shows diffuse enlargement, smooth contour, presence of interlaced fat, and normal vessels. Thymic neoplasia, however, is usually associated with a nodular contour and a heterogeneous appearance with calcification and necrosis. Research so far has shown a limited role for SUV measurements. Data indicate that a SUV_{max} greater than 4.0 may be suggestive of malignancy (thymic carcinoma). However, benign thymic uptake in thymic rebound has overlap with some types of neoplasia (i.e., thymoma).

Other studies may also help distinguish neoplasia from hyperplasia. MRI with chemical shift imaging can show fatty infiltration within thymic rebound, a finding not seen with thymic neoplasia. Additionally, OctreoScan is taken up by thymic tumors but does not accumulate in thymic hyperplasia.

REFERENCES

Jerushalmi J, Frenkel A, Bar-Shalom R, Khoury J, Israel O. Physiologic thymic uptake of 18F-FDG in children and young adults: a PET/CT evaluation of incidence, patterns, and relationship to treatment. *J Nucl Med.* 2009;50(6):849–853.

Nasseri F, Eftekhari F. Clinical and radiologic review of the normal and abnormal thymus: pearls and pitfalls. *Radiographics.* 2010;30(2):413–428.

Case 66

F-18 FDG PET SCAN—MELANOMA

1. d
2. a
3. d
4. c

Discussion

There are numerous clinical and pathologic prognostic criteria for staging melanoma, including the Breslow thickness of the primary tumor, tumor ulceration, the mitotic rate, the extent of local and regional lymph node involvement, and the presence of distant metastases. Other prognostic indicators include serum lactate dehydrogenase (LDH) level. The degree of FDG uptake is not among the prognostic criteria.

Sentinel lymph node biopsy (SLNB) provides the most accurate assessment of sentinel lymph node status, which is the single most important prognostic factor for disease recurrence and survival. SLNB is standard of care for patients without clinical evidence of nodal disease and with a high-risk profile.

FDG PET/CT plays a limited role in the detection of occult nodal metastasis in stage I and II disease because of the small size of the nodal micrometastases and the limited functional resolution of FDG PET. However, in detection of distant metastatic disease in advanced-stage melanoma, FDG PET/CT is highly accurate and has been shown to alter management in ⅓ to ½ of cases of known or suspected metastatic disease. MRI is superior in the detection of brain metastatic disease, and CT of the thorax is better at depicting small pulmonary metastatic lesions, which may be occult on the PET/CT because of low-grade activity and misregistration at the level of the diaphragm.

Studies have reported a correlation between prognosis and anatomic location, showing that lesions of the extremities have a better prognosis than head, neck, and truncal melanomas.

The anterior truncal lesion and hypermetabolic bilateral axillary nodes yield a stage III designation.

REFERENCES

Belhocine TZ, Scott AM, Even-Sapir E, Urbain JL, Essner R. Role of nuclear medicine in the management of cutaneous malignant melanoma. *J Nucl Med*. 2006;47(6):957–967.

Perng P, Marcus C, Subramaniam RM. 18F-FDG PET/CT and melanoma: staging, immune modulation and mutation-targeted therapy assessment, and prognosis. *Am J Roentgenol*. 2015;205(2):259–270.

Case 67

DATSCAN—PARKINSONIAN SYNDROMES

1. c
2. a
3. b
4. a

Discussion

I-123 ioflupane is a radiopharmaceutical that shows the location and concentration of dopamine transporters. The radiotracer, I-123 has a principal photon energy of 159 keV, decays by electron capture, and is well suited to imaging with the gamma camera.

Dopamine transporters are in the presynaptic nigrostriatal axons. The transporters clear and recycle dopamine from the synaptic cleft located in the putamen and caudate nucleus.

Dopamine transporter concentrations are lower in both Parkinson's disease and atypical parkinsonian syndromes, which include multisystem atrophy, progressive supranuclear palsy, dementia with Lewy bodies, and corticobasal degeneration.

I-123 ioflupane single photon-emission computed tomography (SPECT) can help differentiate these syndromes from essential tremor and drug-induced parkinsonism, which have normal dopamine activity.

I-123 ioflupane SPECT has been shown to have a sensitivity and specificity exceeding 90% in differentiating between Parkinson's disease and essential tremor. The scan cannot differentiate between Parkinson's disease and the atypical parkinsonian syndromes.

Abnormal scans typically fall into one of three categories:
- Asymmetric decreased putaminal activity
- Absence of putaminal activity but preserved caudate activity
- Absence of putaminal activity and reduced activity in one or both caudate nuclei

This case illustrates the third pattern of abnormal uptake consistent with parkinsonian syndromes. Normal distribution of the agent shows two symmetric comma- or crescent-shaped areas of activity in the striata (caudate and putamen). Patients with essential tremor have normal scans.

Certain medications (e.g., selegiline, sertraline, citalopram, and paroxetine) can affect the scan, and their presence must be documented and considered before the study.

REFERENCES

Broski Stephen M, Hunt Christopher H, Johnson Geoffrey B, et al. Structural and functional imaging in parkinsonian syndromes. *Radio-Graphics*. 2014;34(5):1273–1292.

Seibyl JP, Kupsch A, Booij J, et al. Individual-reader diagnostic performance and between-reader agreement in assessment of subjects with Parkinsonian syndrome or dementia using 123I-ioflupane injection (DaTscan) imaging. *J Nucl Med*. 2014;55(8):1288–1296.

Case 68

THREE-PHASE BONE SCAN—OSTEOID OSTEOMA (THREE-PHASE BONE SCAN AND CT)

1. d
2. b
3. d
4. c

Discussion

This case demonstrates increased radiotracer activity on all three phases of the bone scan in the proximal left tibia. A dedicated CT scan reveals a cortical-based, centrally lucent nidus with peripheral and central sclerosis consistent with osteoid osteoma.

Osteoid osteoma, a benign tumor of bone, typically occurs in children and adolescents. The classic symptom is that of pain at night alleviated by nonsteroidal antiinflammatory drugs (NSAIDs). Osteoid osteomas often occur in the cortex of the shaft of the long bones, especially the femur and the tibia. These lesions are three-phase (flow (image A), blood pool (image B), and delayed (image C)) positive as a result of hypervascularity. Three-phase-positive findings are nonspecific and require further evaluation with dedicated radiographic imaging. Careful attention must be paid to the clinical history, which may guide the choice of follow-up imaging. In this case we suspected the presence of an osteoid osteoma, so a CT scan was recommended (image D).

Typical radiographic findings include an intracortical nidus, which may show variable amounts of mineralization, accompanied by cortical thickening and reactive sclerosis. The nidus releases prostaglandins (via cyclooxygenase 1 [COX-1] and COX-2), and this, in turn, results in pain. *CT is the modality of choice in locating the nidus.* On CT, the nidus is of low attenuation, well defined, and round or oval in shape. A focus of high

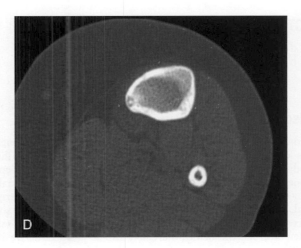

attenuation may be seen centrally, a finding that reflects mineralized osteoid. Adjacent reactive sclerosis may range from mild to extensive periosteal reaction and new bone formation, which may obscure the nidus. Enhancement of a hypervascular nidus may be seen at dynamic CT.

REFERENCES

Chai JW, Hong SH, Choi JY, et al. Radiologic diagnosis of osteoid osteoma: from simple to challenging findings. *Radiographics.* 2010;30(3):737–749.
Laliotis NA, Biacoudi AS, Tsitouridis IA, Petrakis IG, Kirkos JM. Osteoid osteoma of the acetabulum: diagnosis and medical treatment. *J Pediatr Orthop B.* 2017;26(6):565–569.

Case 69

OCTREOSCAN—BRONCHIAL CARCINOID

1. d
2. b
3. c
4. c

Discussion

Bronchopulmonary carcinoids are neuroendocrine neoplasms of the lung. This lesion often presents as a central hilar or perihilar nodule or mass with lobulated borders and an endobronchial component. Carcinoid may be completely or partially endoluminal or may simply abut the airway. Carcinoid tumors may also be peripheral, with no relationship to the bronchus. Tumor may show eccentric, diffuse, or punctate calcification. Because the lesion often obstructs the airway, there may also be postobstructive atelectasis or a clinical history of cough, wheezing, or hemoptysis.

There are two types of carcinoid: typical and atypical. The typical carcinoid is the low-grade malignant lesion with rare extrathoracic metastatic potential. Atypical carcinoid is an intermediate-grade malignancy with metastatic potential. Atypical carcinoid tends to be larger and more peripheral compared with the typical carcinoid.

Carcinoid tumors classically have low-grade uptake on FDG PET like other well-differentiated neuroendocrine tumors. However, well-differentiated carcinoid tumors have somatostatin receptors and can be effectively imaged with In-111 octreotide, a somatostatin analogue. Imaging can be performed at 4, 24, and 48 hours when performing OctreoScan. At 4 hours, approximately 80% to 90% of tumors are visible, and by 24 hours, more are seen as a result of the decreasing background. Early 4-hour imaging is advantageous for imaging of the abdomen/pelvis when there is little physiologic GI activity present.

More recently, somatostatin receptor PET/CT is possible with Ga-68 DOTA-TATE. This newer agent shows superior sensitivity compared with In-111 octreotide, and the combined PET/CT procedure demonstrates increased speed and better detail compared with conventional gamma camera imaging. The technique is also more convenient for the patient because injection and imaging can occur on the same day within a few hours. For both In-111 OctreoScan and Ga-68 DOTA-TATE PET/CT, it is recommended that patients not receive long-acting octreotide for approximately 4 weeks before imaging and that short-acting octreotide be withheld for 24 hours before imaging.

REFERENCES

Benson RE, Rosado-de-Christenson ML, Martínez-Jiménez S, Kunin JR, Pettavel PP. Spectrum of pulmonary neuroendocrine proliferations and neoplasms. *Radiographics*. 2013;33(6):1631–1649.

Granberg D, Sundin A, Janson ET, Öberg K, Skogseid B, Westlin JE. Octreoscan in patients with bronchial carcinoid tumours. *Clin Endocrinol*. 2003;59(6):793–799.

Case 70

MYOCARDIAL PERFUSION STUDY—APICAL MYOCARDIAL INFARCT

1. a
2. d
3. c
4. b

Discussion

This is a case of Tc-99m sestamibi myocardial perfusion study performed at rest and stress (exercise). The images demonstrate a moderately sized fixed defect in the apex, consistent with an infarct. A true perfusion defect should be seen in multiple planes. Defects are usually classified by size (small, moderate, or large) based on the number of segments involved. They are also classified by the intensity of the defect as well as reversibility. This example is severe and not reversible. Multiple perfusion defects involving different vascular territories, if they were present, would be suggestive of multivessel coronary artery disease.

Transient ischemic dilatation is characterized by left ventricular cavity size dilatation on post-stress images compared with the rest images (not seen in this case). This finding is suggestive of triple vessel disease, even if no discrete perfusion defects are identified. It is thought to be related to endocardial stunning or endocardial ischemia. To assess for myocardial viability, an F-18 FDG PET/CT scan should be performed.

In the setting of left bundle branch block (LBBB), an exercise-induced reversible defect may be seen in the septum. This does not occur after pharmacologic stress, and therefore patients with LBBB should not undergo exercise stress testing. It is thought that this may be related to asynchronous relaxation of the septum.

REFERENCES

Inanir S, Caymaz O, Okay T, et al. Tc-99m sestamibi gated SPECT in patients with left bundle branch block. *Clin Nucl Med*. 2001;26(10): 840–846.

Iskander S, Iskandrian AE. Risk assessment using single-photon emission computed tomographic technetium-99m sestamibi imaging. *J Am Coll Cardiol*. 1993;32(1):57–62.

Case 71

GEIGER MULLER COUNTER

1. a
2. a
3. b
4. c

Discussion

This is an image of a Geiger Muller counter. This device is used to measure low levels of radiation, less than 100 mR/hour. This is a gas-filled ionization detector. The output of a Geiger counter is independent of the energy of the incident radiation. It is an all-or-nothing response. These instruments are highly sensitive for the detection of radiation. They are commonly used to survey patients, workers, and work areas for contamination. These instruments should undergo daily battery check, background counting rate check, and constancy check. They should be calibrated at installation, annually, and after service.

The gain switch serves as a multiplier. The actual number of counts detected by the instrument is set by the dial value, which may, then, be multiplied by the gain switch. For example, if the dial needle is set at 2.5k counts per minute (cpm) and the gain switch is set at 10, the actually number of counts measured is 25k cpm.

REFERENCES

Hadley LN. Characteristics of Geiger-Müller Counters. *Proc Okla Acad Sci.* 2015;20:125–126.
Pandey S, Pandey A, Deshmukh M, Shrivastava AK. Role of Geiger Muller counter in modern physics. *J Pure Appl Indust Phys.* 2017;7(5):192–196.

Case 72

I-123 WHOLE-BODY SCAN—LUNG METASTASES FROM THYROID CANCER

1. c
2. a
3. b
4. c

Discussion

This is an I-123 whole-body scan for the assessment of thyroid cancer. The most likely history is that of a palpable thyroid nodule. The other diagnoses would not be iodine avid. There are focal areas of radionuclide uptake in the lungs, consistent with lung metastases. The lung uptake may be diffuse, suggestive of miliary metastatic disease versus focal suggestive of large pulmonary nodules or masses. In the case presented, they are focal. In the past, I-131 was routinely used for whole-body scanning to assess for metastases. At many centers, I-131 has largely been replaced by I-123, which has superior imaging characteristics because of a lower primary photopeak, lower radiation dose to the patient, similar diagnostic quality, and reduced likelihood of stunning compared with I-131. Thyroid stunning may result in decreased uptake of the therapeutic I-131 dose, which may result in decreased therapeutic effect. I-131 has both beta and gamma emissions. The administered I-123 dose is approximately 2 mCi for a whole-body scan. For a dedicated thyroid scan, 200 μCi may be administered. Doses of 15 mCi and 30 mCi are primarily for I-131 therapy for both benign and malignant thyroid diseases.

Before whole-body I-123 imaging, the patient may be taken off levothyroxine to increase the uptake of radiotracer in thyroid tissue. This withdrawal method is poorly tolerated by patients. Therefore most patients will receive two doses of thyrotropin alfa (Thyrogen) injection before radiopharmaceutical injection to stimulate iodine uptake in thyroid tissue. The injections are administered the day before and the day of radiopharmaceutical injection.

REFERENCES

Savir-Baruch B, Barron BJ. Part 6: nuclear medicine–radionuclide therapies. In: *RadTool Nuclear Medicine Flash Facts*. New York: Springer International Publishing; 2017:209–230.

Song HJ, Qiu ZL, Shen CT, Wei WJ, Luo QY. Pulmonary metastases in differentiated thyroid cancer: efficacy of radioiodine therapy and prognostic factors. *Eur J Endocrinol*. 2015;173(3):399–408.

Case 73

BONE SCAN—COMPLEX REGIONAL PAIN SYNDROME

1. a
2. d
3. a
4. d

Discussion

Three-phase bone scan images show increased uptake on three phases to the left forearm and hand, with the delayed images demonstrating increased periarticular uptake distally—findings consistent with complex regional pain syndrome (CRPS), formerly known as *reflex sympathetic dystrophy* (RSD).

CRPS is an exaggerated response to injury, which typically affects a distal extremity (upper or lower), and although the presentation is variable, it is characterized by pain, swelling, skin changes, and vasomotor disturbances. The cause of CRPS is unknown, and the pathophysiology is poorly understood. Precipitating factors include injury, trauma, or surgery to the affected extremity. As well, CRPS may occur after stroke or myocardial infarction.

CRPS diagnosis is made clinically. The classic findings on three-phase bone scan (positive uptake on all three phases with periarticular uptake on delayed imaging) provides the highest diagnostic accuracy but is seen less than 50% of the time. Radiographs may be normal in early disease or may show regional demineralization.

REFERENCES

Birklein F. Complex regional pain syndrome. *J Neurol*. 2005;252(2): 131–138.

Wüppenhorst N, Maier C, Frettlöh J, Pennekamp W, Nicolas V. Sensitivity and specificity of 3-phase bone scintigraphy in the diagnosis of complex regional pain syndrome of the upper extremity. *Clin J Pain*. 2010;26(3):182–189.

Case 74

F-18 FDG PET/CT—PRIMARY CNS LYMPHOMA (PCNSL)

1. b
2. a
3. b
4. a

Discussion

This case demonstrates an FDG-avid intracranial lesion in the left high frontoparietal white matter. Low-grade tumors would not be expected to demonstrate this degree of FDG avidity. Although metastases may be very avid, particularly in tumors such as melanomas, they tend to occur at the gray–white junction, and the history of this patient states that this was a primary CNS malignancy. These are rare tumors accounting for 1% to 5% of all brain tumors. PCNSL lesions tend to be supratentorial in location. The incidence of this tumor is significantly higher in patients who are immunocompromised. Secondary lymphoma of the CNS is more likely to involve the dura and leptomeninges than supratentorial white matter. MRI of the brain with contrast is the primary method for evaluating intracranial lesions, whereas FDG PET/CT is often performed to evaluate for systemic disease. However, these lesions may be incidentally detected in patients with vague complaints for which FDG PET/CT is ordered for a malignancy workup. Almost all of the CNS lymphomas are NHLs. A biopsy is needed for diagnosis as other malignancies may mimic CNS lymphoma on imaging. The literature does support the notion that CNS lymphoma tends to be one of the most FDG-avid tumors in the brain.

REFERENCES

Kosaka N, Tsuchida T, Uematsu H, Kimura H, Okazawa H, Itoh H. 18F-FDG PET of common enhancing malignant brain tumors. *Am J Roentgenol*. 2008 190(6):W365–W369.

Mohile NA, DeAngelis LM, Abrey LE. The utility of body FDG PET in staging primary central nervous system lymphoma. *Neuro Oncol*. 2008;10(2):223–228.

Case 75

THYROID SCAN—SUBACUTE THYROIDITIS

1. d
2. a
3. b
4. c

Discussion

These are pinhole collimator images of the thyroid gland. The left image shows two markers, one denoting the right side of the patient and the other the sternal notch. Both images depict negligible thyroid uptake. The collimator is close to the neck on the right image but further from the patient on the left image. With a history of thyrotoxicosis, neck tenderness, and low radioactive iodine uptake (RAIU), the diagnosis is subacute thyroiditis.

Thyrotoxicosis is defined as hypermetabolism caused by a high level of circulating thyroid hormone, whereas *hyperthyroidism* describes thyrotoxicosis caused by a hyperfunctioning thyroid gland, which could be secondary to such entities as Graves' disease or a toxic multinodular goiter. Thyrotoxicosis may also be caused by inflammation (subacute, silent, postpartum thyroiditis), excess iodine (from drugs or CT contrast agents), or maybe extrathyroidal in etiology (struma ovarii, metastatic thyroid cancer). Thyrotoxicosis resulting from functional thyroid cancer metastases is extremely rare and is mostly caused by follicular cancer.

In a patient with a suppressed thyroid-stimulating hormone (TSH), the RAIU test provides a useful assessment of thyroid function, and in general, the higher the iodine uptake, the more active is the gland. The most useful role of the RAIU test is in determining the etiology of thyrotoxicosis.

Elevated RAIU indicates a hyperfunctioning gland resulting from autonomously functioning thyroid tissue, not under the influence of TSH. Decreased RAIU may be secondary to inflammation (subacute, silent, Hashimoto's, or postpartum thyroiditis), excess iodine, or ectopic thyroid tissue (struma ovarii).

Suppressed RAIU also may result from excessive exogenous thyroid hormone use, also known as *thyroiditis factitia* (or *factitious hyperthyroidism*). This entity is reportedly not uncommon in health care personnel who are able to obtain thyroid hormone, often for the purpose of weight loss. Inadvertent excess thyroid hormone use can also occur from ingestion of certain health food store nutrients that contain desiccated thyroid. A helpful diagnostic tool is the serum thyroglobulin level, which is very low or undetectable in factitious hyperthyroidism. In contrast, the serum thyroglobulin level is generally elevated in endogenous thyrotoxicosis.

REFERENCES

Alfadda AA, Sallam RM, Elawad GE, AlDhukair H, Alyahya MM. Subacute thyroiditis: clinical presentation and long term outcome. *Int J Endocrinol*. 2014;2014(2014):794943.

Intenzo CM, dePapp AE, Jabbour S, Miller JL, Kim SM, Capuzzi DM. Scintigraphic manifestations of thyrotoxicosis. *Radiographics*. 2003;23(4):857–869.

Case 76

F-18 FDG PET CT-LACTATION

1. c
2. c
3. a
4. c

Discussion

Anterior MIP F-18 FDG PET of the chest and upper abdomen shows intense uptake in both breasts as a result of lactation. Mild asymmetry is common.

Increased FDG uptake in lactating breast tissue is thought to be physiologically related to suckling, leading to intracellular trapping of radiotracer in active glandular tissue. Because there is little F-18 FDG excreted into breast milk, the International Commission on Radiologic Protection (ICRP) does not recommend interruption of breastfeeding after F-18 FDG administration. However, it may be suggested that contact between mother and child be limited for 12 hours after injection of F-18 FDG to reduce the radiation dose that the infant receives from external exposure from the mother. It is recommended that the infant be breastfed just before the injection, to maximize the time between the injection and the next feeding.

Another entity that may simulate intense heterogeneous uptake in the breasts is silicone injection granulomas. Free silicone injection performed as a form of breast augmentation was commonly used in the 1950s and 1960s but was banned in by the FDA in 1992 because of safety concerns. This entity may still be seen in immigrants from Asia and South America. The formation of silicone granulomas may occur, causing diffuse inflammation that may show intense FDG uptake.

REFERENCES

Adejolu M, Huo L, Rohren E, Santiago L, Yang WT. False-positive lesions mimicking breast cancer on FDG PET and PET/CT. *Am J Roentgenol.* 2012;198(3):W304–W314.

Dong A, Wang Y, Lu J, Zuo C. Spectrum of the breast lesions with increased 18F-FDG uptake on PET/CT. *Clin Nucl Med.* 2016;41(7):543.

Case 77

THYROID LYMPHOMA

1. b
2. c
3. b
4. d

Discussion

Whole-body F-18 FDG MIP demonstrates a large intensely hypermetabolic mass in the left neck. Biopsy demonstrated NHL of the thyroid in a patient with history of chronic lymphocytic thyroiditis. Graves' disease would be unlikely to cause the symptoms described.

NHL of the thyroid, or primary thyroid lymphoma (PTL), is rare, comprising approximately 5% of all thyroid malignancies and less than 3% of all extranodal lymphomas. Typical presentation is a rapidly enlarging thyroid mass in an elderly female with a history of chronic lymphocytic thyroiditis. The most common histologic subtype is diffuse large B cell lymphoma (DLBCL), comprising up to 70% of cases. The more indolent lymphomas are the subgroup of mucosa-associated lymphoid tissue (MALT) lymphomas comprising approximately 6% to 27% of thyroid lymphomas.

On PET/CT, DLBCL typically demonstrates avid uptake of F-18 FDG within the thyroid and any associated positive cervical lymphadenopathy. The MALT subtype, however, shows low avidity for FDG.

The main differential consideration is anaplastic thyroid carcinoma, which also presents as a rapidly enlarging mass with high FDG uptake. However, anaplastic thyroid carcinoma often is heterogeneous in density, showing calcification, necrosis, and hemorrhage, as well as a propensity for invasion of local structures.

After diagnosis is established, PET/CT is indicated for staging. The Ann Arbor staging system is utilized for PTL. Therapy may include radiation, chemotherapy, and rituximab. Surgery is generally reserved for debulking to relieve airway obstructive symptoms.

REFERENCES

Marcus C, Whitworth PW, Surasi DS, Pai SI, Subramaniam RM. PET/CT in the management of thyroid cancers. *Am J Roentgenol.* 2014;202(6):1316–1329.

Walsh S, Lowery AJ, Evoy D, McDermott EW, Prichard RS. Thyroid lymphoma: recent advances in diagnosis and optimal management strategies. *Oncologist.* 2013;18(9):994–1003.

Case 78

ALZHEIMER'S DISEASE

1. b
2. c
3. c
4. a

Discussion

In this case, there is hypometabolism involving the bilateral parietal and temporal lobes, with relative sparing of the frontal and occipital lobes. Decreased cortical uptake as well involves the posterior cingulate gyrus and the hippocampal regions. This pattern of uptake is classic for Alzheimer's dementia (AD).

PET with FDG is a useful imaging modality for the diagnosis of neurodegenerative disorders, allowing for differentiation among AD, diffuse Lewy body (DLB) disease, and frontotemporal dementia (FTD). FDG is an analogue of glucose, the main energy substrate of the brain. AD, DLB disease, and FTD have shown characteristic patterns of altered cortical glucose metabolism, although with some overlap.

In AD, the classic pattern of hypometabolism consists of involvement of the posterior cingulate gyri, the posterior cingulate precuneus, and the posterior temporal and parietal lobes.

There is often preferential involvement of the posterior cingulate gyrus. The pattern may be symmetric or asymmetric. In more advanced AD, hypometabolism may also involve the frontal lobes, although usually sparing the anterior cingulate.

DLB disease may also show a pattern of bilateral parietal and posterior temporal hypometabolism and posterior cingulate gyral hypometabolism similar to that seen in AD. However, in DLB disease, there can also be associated involvement of the occipital lobes, which are spared in AD. Involvement of the occipital lobes is compatible with the clinical diagnosis of DLB disease.

In FTD, the hypometabolism predominantly involves the frontal and frontal and anterior temporal lobes with involvement of the anterior cingulate gyrus.

REFERENCES

Brown RK, Bohnen NI, Wong KK, Minoshima S, Frey KA. Brain PET in suspected dementia: patterns of altered FDG metabolism. *Radiographics*. 2014;34(3):684–701.

Dukart J, Mueller K, Barthel H, Villringer A, Sabri O, Schroeter ML, Alzheimer's Disease Neuroimaging Initiative. Meta-analysis based SVM classification enables accurate detection of Alzheimer's disease across different clinical centers using FDG-PET and MRI. *Psychiatry Res: Neuroimaging*. 2013;212(3):230–236.

Case 79

BONE SCAN—BREAST CANCER

1. b
2. d
3. c
4. b

Discussion

There is diffuse uptake in the soft tissues of the left breast seen on the anterior planar image only. Focal skeletal uptake is in the sternum, cervical, thoracic, and lumbar spine, which is nonspecific—some of which may be benign and degenerative and some of which may represent metastatic disease. After a dedicated CT scan of the abdomen and pelvis as well as a subsequent F-18 FDG PET/CT, the osseous findings were determined to represent degenerative changes. There was retention of radiotracer in the left arm, which was thought to be related to lymphatic drainage obstruction caused by lymph node involvement in the left axilla.

Differential considerations of extraosseous uptake of bone-seeking radiopharmaceuticals include neoplasm, dystrophic calcification or tissue injury, hypercalcemia, compartmental sequestration, and artifacts related to improper handling or preparation of the tracer or prior radionuclide imaging. In this case, the diffuse asymmetric uptake in the left breast corresponded to locally advanced breast cancer. Uptake in breast cancer may be caused by a combination of factors, including hyperemia, tumor necrosis, pleomorphic calcification, and tumor involvement of the lymphatics causing impaired lymphatic drainage. Benign fibrocystic disease of the breast is not associated with increased uptake on bone scan.

Bone metastases are the most common site of distant disease in breast cancer, accounting for 90% of all metastatic lesions and representing the most common site of initial metastatic involvement. Bone metastases from breast cancer may be osteolytic or osteoblastic. Several studies have shown that FDG PET is superior to bone scintigraphy in detecting lytic and intramedullary metastases. However, FDG PET often fails to show blastic lesions, which are readily seen with bone scintigraphy. In clinical practice, the combination of bone scintigraphy and CT remains the standard imaging combination for staging breast cancer, with FDG PET utilized in equivocal cases.

REFERENCES

Minamimoto R, Loening A, Jamali M, et al Prospective comparison of 99mTc-MDP scintigraphy, combined 18F-NaF and 18F-FDG PET/CT, and whole-body MRI in patients with breast and prostate cancer. *J Nucl Med.* 2015;56(12):1862–1868.

Wale DJ, Wong KK, Savas H, Kandathil A, Piert M, Brown RK. Extraosseous findings on bone scintigraphy using fusion SPECT/CT and correlative imaging. *Am J Roentgenol.* 2015;205(1):160–172.

Case 80

QC—FREE TC-99M PERTECHNETATE

1. c
2. a
3. d
4. b

Discussion

Anterior whole-body scintigraphy shows oral and gastric activity. These findings are caused by free pertechnetate that distributes to the stomach, salivary glands, and thyroid gland. In this case, the activity is most intense in the stomach and oral cavity, probably within the saliva.

Tc-99m radiopharmaceuticals are typically made from commercially available kits that contain a multidose reaction vial containing stannous ion (the reducing agent) and the nonradioactive pharmaceutical to be labeled. The vial is flushed with nitrogen to prevent oxygen from interfering with the reaction. Tc-99m is added to the reaction vial. However, if excessive air is introduced into the reaction vial, the air may cause oxidation and breakdown of the radiolabeled compound with release of free Tc-99m pertechnetate. Testing of the labeled radiopharmaceutical for radiochemical purity can be performed with radiochromatography to assess for excess free pertechnetate. This must be done before injection of the radiopharmaceutical. No further workup is required for this patient because the classic imaging findings are diagnostic of free pertechnetate.

REFERENCES

Gentili A, Miron SD, Adler LP. Review of some common artifacts in nuclear medicine. *Clin Nucl Med*. 1994;19(2):138–143.

Gnanasegaran G, Cook G, Adamson K, Fogelman I. Patterns, variants, artifacts, and pitfalls in conventional radionuclide bone imaging and SPECT/CT. *Semin Nucl Med*. 2009;39(6):380–395.

Case 81

CROSSED CEREBELLAR DIASCHISIS

1. b
2. b
3. c
4. d

Discussion

This is a case of crossed cerebellar diaschisis. The diagnosis refers to decreased perfusion or metabolism contralateral to a supratentorial abnormality. For example, a right middle cerebral artery (MCA) infarct may cause a decrease in radiotracer uptake in the left cerebellar hemisphere. The supratentorial abnormality may be a result of tumor, encephalomalacia, postoperative change, or infarct, to name a few. This abnormality may manifest shortly after the onset of the supratentorial abnormality. This finding is thought to be related to dysfunction of the cerebropontocerebellar pathways. The degree of cerebellar hypo(perfusion) metabolism is directly proportion to the degree of supratentorial insult. If there is diffuse brain injury, this pattern may not be seen.

This is an F-18 FDG PET brain scan. Brain SPECT CT (Tc-99m ethyl cysteinate dimer [ECD] or hexamethylpropyleneamine oxime [HMPAO]) of the brain would show a similar finding. One way to decipher whether it is a perfusion scan or a metabolic scan is to look for uptake in the extraocular muscles (will be avid on an FDG PET scan, not on a perfusion scan).

REFERENCES

Alavi A, Mirot A, Newberg A, Alves W. Fluorine-18-FDG evaluation of crossed cerebellar diaschisis in head injury. *J Nucl Med*. 1997;38(11):1717.
Komaba Y, Mishina M, Utsumi K, Katayama Y, Kobayashi S, Mori O. Crossed cerebellar diaschisis in patients with cortical infarction. *Stroke*. 2004;35(2):472–476.

Case 82

TC-99M RBC SCAN—SPLENOSIS

1. b
2. b
3. d
4. a

Discussion

This is a Tc-99m RBC scan which demonstrates radiotracer uptake outside the vascular pool. The foci of uptake did not move ante or retrograde on dynamic imaging (images not shown). Hence, a SPECT CT was performed, and it localized the uptake in soft tissue outside the bowel lumen (not shown). The lack of movement would negate the diagnosis of GI bleed. Concurrent CT of the abdomen (image B) demonstrated multiple soft tissue nodules dispersed within the abdomen. The spleen was not visualized. When questioned, the patient gave a history of

prior trauma. The most common etiologies for splenosis are trauma and hematologic conditions. Splenosis most commonly occurs within the abdomen but may be found within the chest. Numerous case reports describing erroneous diagnoses of metastases or neoplasia in patients with splenosis have been published. Tc-99m RBC is an effective method for confirming the diagnosis of splenosis. Tc-99m SC is most commonly used for characterization of abdominal lesions thought to represent splenic tissue (Figures 82-1A and 82-1B).

REFERENCES

Esguerra V, Diaz P. Malignancy mimic: an unexpected consequence of an abdominal gun shot wound. In: *B38. Pleural Disease: Case Reports.* New York: American Thoracic Society; 2016: A3330–A3330.

Hagan I, Hopkins R, Lyburn I. Superior demonstration of splenosis by heat-denatured Tc-99m red blood cell scintigraphy compared with Tc-99m sulfur colloid scintigraphy. *Clin Nucl Med.* 2006;31(8):463–466.

Case 83

QUALITY CONTROL—FOUR-QUADRANT BAR PHANTOM

1. b
2. b
3. d
4. b

Discussion

This is a four-quadrant bar phantom image, which is performed weekly as a part of normal quality control assessment of gamma cameras. This image is used to assess for linearity and spatial resolution. This is a qualitative assessment. Quantitative assessment may be performed at acceptance and, in some instances, annually. Each quadrant is composed of alternating lead bars and radiolucent plastic strips 2, 2.5, 3, and 4 mm in width. To obtain the image, the phantom is placed on the collimator, with a large uniform source placed on top of it, and 5 to 10 million count transmission images are acquired. The qualitative assessment consists of visually determining in which quadrants one can clearly discern separation between bars and air (spatial resolution) and whether the lines are straight (linearity). The rule of thumb is that the bars discerned should measure at 60% of the quantitative spatial resolution value (measured in millimeters). The two quadrants with the largest widths should be easily discernable as discrete lines. The 2.5-mm quadrant should also largely be visible. Discrete lines should be straight in all quadrants.

REFERENCE

Sokole EB, Płachcínska A, Britten A, Georgosopoulou ML, Tindale W, Klett R. Routine quality control recommendations for nuclear medicine instrumentation. *Eur J Nucl Med Mol Imaging*. 2010;37(3):662–671.

Case 84

CARDIAC PET SCANS—HIBERNATING MYOCARDIUM

1. c
2. c
3. b
4. b

Discussion

This is a cardiac PET scan composed of a perfusion scan performed at rest and a follow-up FDG scan. The imaging findings are a large perfusion defect in the inferior and inferior septal wall that takes up glucose on subsequent FDG images compatible with viable hibernating myocardium. The perfusion scan is performed first because of the short half-life of either Rb82 or NH3 ammonia. This allows for subsequent imaging with FDG on the same day. The scan is performed to evaluate for myocardial viability in a fixed perfusion defect associated with contractile dysfunction. Normal, healthy myocardium preferentially utilizes fatty acids for metabolism. Hibernating myocardium, however, switches to glucose metabolism, which may be greater than that in the adjacent healthy myocardium. This is referred to as *metabolic perfusion mismatch*. A defect that demonstrates no evidence of perfusion or glucose metabolism is thought to represent a scar. The reason to perform this test is that patients with hibernating myocardium are thought to benefit from revascularization compared with those with scar formation.

Patient preparation for the FDG portion of the examination is more elaborate than most other PET/CT studies. The goal is to induce an environment where the myocardium will preferentially utilize glucose over fatty acids. This is usually done by giving the patient a glucose load after a fasting period. This induces an insulin response, which reduces fatty acid levels. Although glucose loading may be done with intravenous administration, most places utilize oral glucose loading ranging from 25 to 100 mg. To induce the drop in glucose levels, IV insulin may be added to the regimen. Patients with diabetes may not produce an insulin response and therefore benefit from IV insulin administration routinely.

REFERENCES

Abraham A, Nichol G, Williams KA, et al. 18F-FDG PET imaging of myocardial viability in an experienced center with access to 18F-FDG and integration with clinical management teams: the Ottawa-FIVE substudy of the PARR 2 trial. *J Nucl Med.* 2010;51(4):567–574.

Sheikine Y, Di Carli MF. Integrated PET/CT in the assessment of etiology and viability in ischemic heart failure. *Curr Heart Fail Rep.* 2008;5(3):136–142.

Case 85

PET SCAN—SARCOIDOSIS

1. a
2. b
3. a
4. d

Discussion

This is an FDG PET scan that demonstrates diffuse FDG-avid adenopathy in the chest and abdomen. Activity projecting over the liver on MIP images localized to lymph nodes on cross-sectional images. The adenopathy in the chest has a distribution that is suggestive of sarcoidosis. A clinical history of interstitial lung disease is also suggestive of the diagnosis. However, lymphoma and underlying inflammatory disease may have a similar appearance on F-18 FDG PET/CT.

Sarcoidosis is a chronic disease of unknown etiology characterized by the formation of noncaseating granulomas in any organ of the body. The most common organs involved include lung, liver, spleen, and skin. Bone lesions may also be seen. Common clinical symptoms include fever, weight loss, fatigue, and malaise. Incidental diagnoses based on skin lesions, abnormal results on chest radiography performed for other reasons, eye complaints, or cardiac events are less common. Pulmonary findings include mediastinal and hilar adenopathy as well as interstitial lung parenchymal findings. There are four classifications based on radiographic findings.

Type I: Hilar and mediastinal adenopathy without lung findings

Type II: Hilar and mediastinal adenopathy and interstitial lung disease

Type III: Diffuse pulmonary disease without evidence of mediastinal or hilar adenopathy

Type IV: Pulmonary fibrosis

Sarcoidosis may spontaneously resolve or progressively worsen with time. Diagnosis is confirmed with biopsy. Steroids are the mainstay of therapy to reduce inflammation. F-18 FDG PET/CT may be used to aid in the diagnosis as well as assess treatment response.

REFERENCES

Incerti E, Cremona G, Gajate AMS, et al. 18F-FDG PET as treatment guide in patients with sarcoidosis. *J Nucl Med.* 2015;56(suppl 3):1730.

Soussan M, Augier A, Brillet PY, Weinmann P, Valeyre D. Functional imaging in extrapulmonary sarcoidosis: FDG-PET/CT and MR features. *Clin Nucl Med.* 2014;39(2):e146–e159.

Case 86

PANCREATIC CANCER

1. a
2. a
3. d
4. d

Discussion

Images from the PET/CT show focal, intense uptake in the pancreatic head and neck corresponding with a heterogeneously enhancing mass. No other uptake is evident. Further evaluation and biopsy with endoscopic US revealed pancreatic adenocarcinoma.

Pancreatic tumors show variable uptake on FDG PET, depending on tumor histology and size. Islet cell tumors of the pancreas characteristically have low-grade activity on FDG PET, whereas the other tumors listed can show intense activity.

Several studies have shown that FDG PET/CT is most useful in initial staging of disease because of its ability to detect distant metastatic disease, thus altering patient management and avoiding unnecessary surgery. FDG PET/CT, however, is not indicated for determining tumor resectability because of its limited spatial resolution. Contrast-enhanced CT is superior in delineating involvement of vascular structures and determining resectability.

REFERENCES

Asagi A, Ohta K, Nasu J, et al. Utility of contrast-enhanced FDG-PET/CT in the clinical management of pancreatic cancer: impact on diagnosis, staging, evaluation of treatment response, and detection of recurrence. *Pancreas*. 2013;42(1):11–19.

Wang XY, Yang F, Jin C, Fu DL. Utility of PET/CT in diagnosis, staging, assessment of resectability and metabolic response of pancreatic cancer. *World J Gastroenterol*. 2014;20(42):15580.

Case 87

F-18 FDG PET/CT SCAN—WARTHIN'S TUMOR

1. d
2. d
3. a
4. b

Discussion

The fused PET/CT image shows bilateral, multifocal, rounded hypermetabolic activity in the parotid glands.

Several retrospective studies have shown that FDG-positive parotid incidentalomas occur in approximately 0.3% to 0.4% of PET/CT scans. The majority of these lesions are benign, most commonly benign mixed tumor and Warthin's tumor. In a small percentage of cases the lesions may be malignant. Studies suggest patients with a prior history of lymphoma have a higher risk of parotid malignancy. PET/CT is unable to differentiate benign lesions from malignant parotid lesions on the basis of SUV_{max}.

Warthin's tumor is a benign tumor arising from salivary lymphoid tissue in intraparotid and periparotid nodes. It is the most common mass arising in the parotid tail, superficial to the angle of the mandible. There is a strong association with smoking—90% of patients with Warthin's tumor have a smoking history. Approximately 20% of the tumors are multifocal. Additionally, there is a reported association with Epstein-Barr virus in those with multifocal, bilateral disease.

Although frequently benign, parotid incidentalomas may require further investigation and can often be sampled via US guidance. MRI imaging may be necessary for preoperative planning for larger lesions or for those lesions located in the deep portion of the gland (Figure 87-1).

REFERENCES

Britt CJ, Stein AP, Patel PN, Harari PM, Hartig GK. Incidental parotid neoplasms: pathology and prevalence. *Otolaryngol Head Neck Surg.* 2015;153(4):566–568.

Seo YL, Yoon DY, Baek S, et al. Incidental focal FDG uptake in the parotid glands on PET/CT in patients with head and neck malignancy. *Eur Radiol.* 2015;25(1):171–177.

Case 88

BONE SCAN—STERNAL UPTAKE IN BREAST CANCER

1. b
2. c
3. a
4. d

Discussion

This is a bone scan performed on a patient with breast cancer for evaluation of osseous metastases. There is focal uptake in the mid-sternum. Focal uptake in the sternum is most often seen at the sternomanubrial joint related to degenerative/physiologic changes. This activity does not localize to the sternomanubrial joint but to the body of the sternum. Although isolated lesions seen on bone scan in patients with history of malignancy are more likely to represent benign disease, focal uptake in the sternum in a patient with breast cancer has an approximately 80% chance of representing metastases. Bone is the most common site of metastases in breast cancer. Up to 40% of patients may only have a single site of bone metastases.

REFERENCES

Fontanella C, Fanotto V, Rihawi K, Aprile G, Puglisi F. Skeletal metastases from breast cancer: pathogenesis of bone tropism and treatment strategy. *Clin Exp Metastasis*. 2015;32(8):819–833.

Kwai AH, Stomper PC, Kaplan WD. Clinical significance of isolated scintigraphic sternal lesions in patients with breast cancer. *J Nucl Med*. 1988;29(3):324–328.

Case 89

ADRENAL METASTASES

1. b
2. d
3. b
4. c

Discussion

The etiology of hypermetabolic (SUV_{max} greater than or equal to that of the liver) bilateral adrenal gland masses is highly dependent on clinical history.

Metastases to the adrenal glands are common in patients who have a history of malignant disease, and tumors of the lung, breast, melanoma, kidney, colon, esophagus, pancreas, liver, and stomach commonly metastasize to the adrenal gland. Bilateral adrenal metastatic involvement is more common than unilateral. Although PET/CT has high sensitivity and specificity for detection of adrenal metastasis, which are typically FDG avid, in patients with malignancy approximately 16% of benign adrenal lesions may show false-positive FDG uptake relative to the background, and false-negative findings may be seen in adrenal metastasis with hemorrhage or necrosis, small metastatic nodules (<1 cm), and metastases from adenocarcinoma in situ of lung or carcinoid tumors.

Pheochromocytomas are also hypermetabolic on FDG PET/CT. Several genetic syndromes are associated with pheochromocytomas, such as multiple endocrine neoplasia type 2A (MEN 2A), MEN 2B, Von Hippel-Lindau disease, and neurofibromatosis type 1 (NF1). These patients present with bilateral lesions more commonly compared with patients with sporadic pheochromocytoma.

Adrenal tuberculosis is usually bilateral and, in the acute phase, highly FDG avid. In the acute phase, CT may show masslike enlargement of the adrenal glands with peripheral rim enhancement and low attenuation in the center, reflecting necrosis. Adrenal tuberculosis is the major cause of primary adrenal insufficiency (Addison's disease) in the developing countries, and patients may present with an addisonian-like clinical picture, including, fatigue, weakness, anorexia, nausea and vomiting, and changes in skin pigmentation.

REFERENCES

Dong A, Cui Y, Wang Y, Zuo C, Bai Y. 18F-FDG PET/CT of adrenal lesions. *Am J Roentgenol.* 2014;203(2):245–252.

Shin YR, Kim KA. Imaging features of various adrenal neoplastic lesions on radiologic and nuclear medicine imaging. *Am J Roentgenol.* 2015;205(3):554–563.

Case 90

F-18 FDG PET/CT—GASTRIC CANCER

1. c
2. d
3. a
4. d

Discussion

The CT image at the level of the stomach showed marked diffuse thickening of the anterior wall, with diffuse soft tissue haziness extending from the wall into the adjacent peritoneum, consistent with abnormal hypermetabolic activity on F-18 FDG PET. Biopsy findings were consistent with adenocarcinoma, intestinal type. No other uptake was noted on the whole-body MIP to indicate metastatic disease.

Stomach cancer remains the second most common cancer worldwide. In Asian countries, such as Korea, China, and Japan, as well as in many developing countries, gastric cancer is the most prevalent malignant neoplasm and the leading cause of cancer death. Risk factors include infection with *Helicobacter pylori*, pernicious anemia, and a diet heavy in nitrites and nitrates. In primary tumor detection, FDG uptake in gastric adenocarcinoma is variable, depending on the histologic subtype. The intestinal subtype typically shows higher SUV_{max} than the diffuse subtypes (mucinous carcinoma and signet ring cell carcinoma), which tend to show significantly lower FDG uptake. The size of the tumor also contributes significantly to FDG-PET detection of primary tumors with an increased number of locally advanced gastric cancers detectable by PET/CT compared with early gastric cancers.

As with other malignancies, the major advantage of FDG PET over anatomic imaging modalities is its ability to help detect distant solid organ metastases. Metastases to the liver, lungs, adrenal glands, and ovaries can be readily identified at FDG PET. Peritoneal disease, however, may not be as readily detected by PET/CT because of the small size of the peritoneal lesions.

REFERENCES

Lim JS, Yun MJ, Kim MJ, et al. CT and PET in stomach cancer: preoperative staging and monitoring of response to therapy. *Radiographics*. 2006;26(1):143–155.

Stahl A, Ott K, Weber W, et al. FDG PET imaging of locally advanced gastric carcinomas correlation with endoscopic and histopathological findings. *Eur J Nucl Med Mol Imaging*. 2003;30(2):288–295.

Case 91

FDG PET CT—DISCITIS/OSTEOMYELITIS WITH EPIDURAL ABSCESS

1. b
2. b
3. c
4. a

Discussion

This is a case of an oncologic FDG PET being performed on a patient with history of head and neck cancer. The patient, disease free for 3 years, came in with complaints of new neck pain. The clinical team was concerned about recurrence of the neoplasm and ordered an outpatient FDG PET scan. FDG PET scans of the chest, abdomen, and pelvis did not reveal FDG-avid disease; however, focal activity was seen in the neck extending into the cervical spinal canal. Upon further questioning, patient revealed recent ingestion of a chicken bone that got stuck in the throat but then cleared spontaneously. An emergent MRI of the cervical spine was performed, and it revealed findings consistent with discitis/osteomyelitis with an epidural abscess. Because some neurologic deficits were revealed on examination, the patient was taken to the operating room (OR) for decompression. The findings in the OR were consistent with the radiologic diagnosis.

F-18 FDG PET/CT is often utilized to assess for underlying infection. If the findings are negative, the presence of an infection is essentially ruled out. When the findings are positive, they may be confounded by focal inflammation or trauma. The protocol, including patient preparation for evaluating for infection, is identical to FDG PET being performed for oncologic purposes.

When evaluating for osteomyelitis of the spine, Ga-67 with SPECT CT may also be considered. In-111 WBC scan is not preferred over Ga-67 because of high false-negative rates in the spine. Three-phase bones scans are nonspecific and frequently require follow-up imaging with the other techniques. If there is an urgent need to diagnose an infection, F-18 FDG PET/CT is the imaging modality of choice because of its 1-day imaging protocols compared with those of the other techniques.

REFERENCES

Meller J, Sahlmann CO, Scheel AK. 18F-FDG PET and PET/CT in fever of unknown origin. *J Nucl Med*. 2007;48(1):35–45.

Strobel K, Stumpe KD. PET/CT in musculoskeletal infection. In: *Seminars in Musculoskeletal Radiology*. New York: Thieme Medical Publishers; 2007;11(4):353–364.

Case 92

VENTRICULOPERITONEAL SHUNT CATHETER EVALUATION/CISTERNOGRAM—OBSTRUCTED

1. b
2. a
3. a
4. b

Discussion

This case demonstrates dynamic images of a ventriculoperitoneal shunt catheter evaluation (Image A). Image B comprises static images of the head and abdomen immediately after the dynamic phase. There is no evidence of radiotracer transit into the abdomen. The port is accessed by using sterile technique. The radiopharmaceutical is injected with the patient under the camera, and imaging is begun immediately before injection. The radiopharmaceuticals most commonly used include In-111 DTPA and Tc-99m DTPA. In-111 DTPA is expensive and exposes the patient to significant amounts of radiation; hence, many Nuclear Medicine departments routinely use Tc-99m DTPA.

The $t\frac{1}{2}$ emptying time should be less than 10 minutes. In this case, the curve is relatively flat, consistent with no spontaneous clearing. If there is no immediate drainage, the patient is asked to ambulate, and repeat imaging of the abdomen is performed at 10 minutes to look for dispersal of radiotracer within the peritoneal cavity. If there is dispersal, the catheter is thought to be obstructed because of the position of the patient. If there is no dispersal at 10 minutes and 2 hours, findings are consistent with complete obstruction.

REFERENCES

Kale HA, Muthukrishnan A, Hegde SV, Agarwal V. Intracranial perishunt catheter fluid collections with edema, a sign of shunt malfunction: correlation of CT/MRI and nuclear medicine findings. *AJNR Am J Neuroradiol.* 2017;38(9):1754–1757.

Tsai SY, Wang SI, Shiau YC, Yang LH, Wu YW. The clinical value of radionuclide shuntography in hydrocephalic adult patients with suspected ventriculo-peritoneal shunt malfunction. *J Nucl Med.* 2016;57(suppl 2):1774.

Case 93

PET SCAN—RIGHT HUMERAL ENCHONDROMA

1. b
2. d
3. c
4. a

Discussion

In this case, there is mild diffuse uptake in the proximal metaphysis of the right humerus, corresponding to an ill-defined area of mild radiolucency with subtle, ring-and-arc chondroid matrix at the anterior margin of the lesion. There is no endosteal scalloping or sclerotic margin. No other aggressive feature noted. SUV_{max} is 2.2. Finding is consistent with a benign enchondroma.

The SUV_{max} of a primary bone tumor on an FDG PET scan does not necessarily predict malignant potential. For example, low-grade malignant chondrosarcoma may show very low uptake with SUV_{max}, and this may overlap with benign lesions, such as hemangioma, enchondroma, intraosseous lipoma, and osteochondroma, which also consistently show low-grade uptake. Conversely, a benign bone tumor, such as a giant cell tumor, may be highly FDG avid. Thus, the morphologic assessment of the bone lesion (aggressive or nonaggressive) on the CT portion of the scan is important in determining whether biopsy of the lesion should be performed to assess its malignant potential. CT characteristics of an aggressive lesion include a wide zone of transition between the lesion and normal bone; periosteal reaction that is multilayered, lamellated, or perpendicular to the bone; and cortical interruption or destruction, with an associated soft tissue mass. A thick sclerotic margin implies a chronic, long-standing process that is more likely to be benign.

REFERENCES

Costelloe CM, Chuang HH, Madewell JE. FDG PET/CT of primary bone tumors. *Am J Roentgenol*. 2014;202(6):W521–W531.

Feldman F, Van Heertum R, Saxena C, Parisien M. 18FDG-PET applications for cartilage neoplasms. *Skeletal Radiol*. 2005;34(7):367–374.

Case 94

THYROID PROBE SYSTEM

1. c
2. c
3. c
4. d

Discussion

This is an image of a thyroid probe. It is used to measure thyroid uptake of iodine radiotracers. The probe typically consists of a sodium iodide crystal with a cone shaped (diverging) collimator. The sodium iodide crystal measures 5 cm in diameter and thickness. Photomultiplier tubes are placed adjacent to the crystal. It is important to place the probe close to the patient's neck to exclude extraneous radiation from other patients. The probe should be placed at a standard distance from the patient to maintain quantitative integrity for the Nuclear Medicine laboratory.

Thyroid uptake measurements consist of background or room uptake and thigh uptake, which measure activity in extrathyroidal tissues; thyroid uptake; and standard thyroid phantom uptake (usually measured before administration of iodine). A known dose is placed in a plastic phantom and counts obtained. The dose is ingested by the patient and neck counts are acquired at 4 hours and/or 24 hours after ingestion and corrected for decay and background. The percent uptake is: Neck counts ÷ Phantom counts ≡ Percent uptake. Normal thyroid uptake varies by laboratories but generally ranges from 15% to 30%.

REFERENCES

Biersack H, Freeman L. *Clinical Nuclear Medicine*. Berlin, Germany: Springer; 2007.

Sokole EB, Płachcińska A, Britten A, Georgosopoulou ML, Tindale W, Klett R. Routine quality control recommendations for nuclear medicine instrumentation. *Eur J Nucl Med Mol Imaging*. 2010;37(3):662–671.

Case 95

MO-99/TC-99 GENERATOR

1. d
2. c
3. b
4. b

Discussion

The Mo-99/Tc-99 generator is the workhorse of the Nuclear Medicine department. Some clinical departments will have their own generators, whereas others will order unit doses from larger central pharmacies. Mo-99 is produced by fission of uranium-235 (U-235). Mo-99 is then chemically purified and passed on to an aluminum oxide (Al_2O_3) ion exchange column. Over time Mo-99 (parent compound) decays into Tc-99m. The maximum buildup of Tc-99m occurs at 23 hours. This is a dynamic environment where Tc-99m decays into stable Tc-99 overtime. Although Tc-99 is not an impurity, it may interfere with labeling efficiency. The most common radionuclide impurity is Mo-99 in an eluate.

The NRC limit is 0.15 μCi per 1 mCi of Tc-99m (0.3 μCi per 2 mCi of Tc-99m) in a dose to be administered.

There are two main generator systems, wet and dry. Wet systems have a built-in reservoir of saline, whereas dry systems require placing a sterile saline vial onto the system for elution. The Al_2O_3 column packing material may be found in the eluate. Colorimetric testing can assess for this chemical impurity. Excess Al_2O_3 may result in increased lung uptake with Tc-99m SC or liver uptake with Tc-99m MDP. Radiochemical impurity evaluates the chemical form of Tc-99m. The ideal chemical form has a valence state of +7. The United States Pharmacopeia standard is that a generator eluate should contain 95% or greater activity in the +7 state. This can be evaluated by thin layer chromatography. Pyrogenicity is not commonly assessed.

REFERENCE

Chandra R, Rahmim A. *Nuclear Medicine Physics: The Basics*. New York: Lippincott Williams & Wilkins; 2017.

Case 96

F-18 FDG PET—MAI BONE INFECTION

1. d
2. d
3. b
4. d

Discussion

Multiple images from the initial FDG PET/CT of the whole body showed intensely hypermetabolic mixed lytic and sclerotic lesions in the axial and appendicular skeleton. Biopsy of the right wrist showed *Mycobacterium avium* complex infection. The patient was treated with isoniazid, rifampin, ethambutol, and pyrazinamide, and repeat imaging 4 months later showed overall decrease in uptake in multiple lesions. There was no radiographic evidence of bony exostosis to suggest multiple hereditary exostosis.

FDG uptake in tumor, infection, and inflammation is facilitated by upregulation of glucose transporters (in particular GLUT1). Also, in inflammatory conditions, the affinity of glucose transporters for deoxyglucose is increased by various cytokines, a phenomenon not observed in tumor. Leukocytes, which include neutrophils, monocytes, macrophages, and lymphocytes, all demonstrate increased uptake in infection/inflammation.

According to the Society of Nuclear Medicine and Molecular Imaging (SNMMI) and the European Association of Nuclear Medicine (EANM), the major indications for F-18 FDG PET/CT in infection and inflammation are sarcoidosis, peripheral bone osteomyelitis (non-postoperative, nondiabetic foot), suspected spine infection (spondylodiskitis or vertebral osteomyelitis, non-postoperative); evaluation of fever of unknown origin (FUO), metastatic infection, and high-risk patients with bacteremia, and primary evaluation of vasculitides (e.g., giant cell arteritis).

REFERENCES

Lin KH, Wang JH, Peng NJ. Disseminated nontuberculous mycobacterial infection mimic metastases on PET/CT scan. *Clini Nuclear Med*. 2003;3(4): 276–277.

Palestro CJ. FDG-PET in musculoskeletal infections. *Semin Nucl Med* 2013;43(5):367–376.

Case 97

TC-99M RBC SCAN—HEMANGIOMA

1. c
2. b
3. a
4. c

Discussion

This is a tagged RBC scan performed for the evaluation of a liver lesion. Persistent uptake in the vascular pool should clue one in that this is a RBC scan. This test is performed to determine whether a liver lesion seen on cross-sectional imaging represents a hemangioma. The radiotracer tends to accumulate in this lesions after initial uptake in the liver and persists as the normal background liver clears. This has a high sensitivity and specificity. As the CT and MRI imaging technologies have advanced, the need for this test has declined. However, it is a good technique to problem solve if there is still a question of exact diagnosis after anatomic evaluation has been performed. The most common reason for a false-negative result is the small size of the primary lesion.

REFERENCES

Dong H, Zhang Z, Guo Y, Zhang H, Xu W. The application of technetium-99m-red blood cell scintigraphy in the diagnosis of orbital cavernous hemangioma. *Nucl Med Commun*. 2017;38(9):744.

Roy SG, Karunanithi S, Agarwal KK, Bal C, Kumar R. Importance of SPECT/CT in detecting multiple hemangiomas on 99mTc-labeled RBC blood pool scintigraphy. *Clin Nucl Med*. 2015;40(4):345–346.

Case 98

PET SCAN—CERVICAL CANCER

1. b
2. c
3. a
4. d

Discussion

PET/CT is the modality of choice for initial staging of cervical cancer and for the management of recurrent disease. The main benefit of PET/CT is in the detection of locoregional and distant nodal metastases and the subsequent change in management. The identification of involved nodes facilitates radiation therapy planning.

MRI and contrast-enhanced CT are better for evaluating the extent of the primary lesion.

One-third of patients have disease recurrence within 2 years. Studies have shown that PET/CT has high accuracy for the detection of locally recurrent disease and distant metastatic disease. Current recommendations for imaging surveillance, however, are based on history and physical examination. If recurrent disease is suspected on the basis of symptoms or examination, imaging is then recommended to evaluate the extent of disease, and a biopsy specimen should be obtained for analysis to confirm recurrence. PET/CT scanning is then usually performed before definitive radiation or exenterative surgery to identify distant disease that may alter management.

The major risk factor for development of cervical cancer is infection with human papilloma virus (HPV), particularly HPV-16 and HPV-18. Other risk factors also include early onset of sexual activity, high number of sexual partners, cigarette smoking, immunosuppression, and history of sexually transmitted diseases (STDs).

Staging of cervical cancer according to the TNM (tumor–node–metastasis) staging system is as follows:
- Stage I: T1 and N0, M0
- Stage II: T2 and N0, M0
- Stage III: T3 and any N, M0
- Stage IV: T4 and any N, any M

Additionally,
- T1: Confined to uterus
- T2: Invades beyond uterus, but not to pelvic wall or lower one-third of vagina
- T3: Extends to pelvic wall or lower one-third of vagina and/or causes hydronephrosis or renal failure
- T4: Invades bladder/rectum and/or extends beyond true pelvis

In performing PET/CT for cervical cancer staging, techniques to decrease the activity from the urinary bladder, which may obscure the primary lesion and confound interpretation of adjacent pelvic activity, varies among institutions. Bladder catheterization, repeat imaging after voiding, and diuretic protocols have been utilized.

REFERENCES

Papadopoulou I, Stewart V, Barwick TD, et al. Post-radiation therapy imaging appearances in cervical carcinoma. *Radiographics*. 2016;36(2):538–553.

Salani R, Khanna N, Frimer M, Bristow RE, Chen LM. An update on post-treatment surveillance and diagnosis of recurrence in women with gynecologic malignancies: Society of Gynecologic Oncology (SGO) recommendations. *Gynecol Oncol*. 2017;146(1):3–10.

Case 99

PET—BRAIN AMYLOID

1. c
2. a
3. c
4. c

Discussion

The normal scan on the left (Image A) shows low-level uptake limited to the white matter tracts. The abnormal positive scan on the right (Image B) shows extensive uptake in cortical gray matter in addition to white matter, resulting in loss of gray matter–white matter differentiation.

AD is the most common cause of dementia. Neurofibrillary tangles and beta amyloid plaques are the two neuropathologic hallmarks of AD. Amyloid plaques are found between the neurons and neurofibrillary tangles are found within neurons and both can be identified postmortem by using special stains.

The first specific tracer for beta amyloid, carbon-11 (C-11)–labeled Pittsburgh Compound B (PiB), was based on one of these histopathologic stains, thioflavin T. The C-11 PiB radiopharmaceutical binds to cortical gray matter plaques in 90% of patients with AD. However, the short half-life (20 minutes) of the C-11 isotope limits the clinical utility of the C-11 PiB compound, requiring an on-site cyclotron, precluding widespread distribution and clinical application. Recently, a second generation of amyloid tracers labeled with F-18 has been developed, allowing for widespread distribution because of the longer half-life of F-18 (110 minutes). There are now three FDA-approved F-18 tracers, which include florbetapir (Amyvid, Eli Lilly), flutemetamol (Vizamyl, GE Healthcare), and florbetaben (NeuraCeq, Piramal Pharma).

Published appropriate use criteria (AUC) for amyloid PET recommends the following imaging indications:

1. Persistent or progressive unexplained MCI
2. Clinical criteria for possible AD satisfied, but the clinical presentation is atypical

3. Patients with progressive dementia and a typical early age of onset (defined as age 65 years or less)

Amyloid imaging is considered *inappropriate* in the following cases:

1. Patients with clinical criteria for probable AD with typical age of onset
2. Determination of dementia severity
3. Asymptomatic individuals
4. Nonmedical use (e.g., legal, insurance coverage, or employment screening)

There is no specific preparation for patients before imaging. Unlike F-18 FDG PET/CT imaging, patients are not required to be NPO (nothing by mouth). Sedation may be considered in patients who are unable to hold still or tolerate the procedure.

The scans are generally read in a binary fashion—negative or positive. Because amyloid plaques may be present in patients who are cognitively normal, a positive scan is positive for amyloid plaque presence and is not diagnostic of disease (AD). A negative scan rules out AD with a high degree of certainty.

REFERENCES

Johnson KA, Minoshima S, Bohnen NI, et al. Update on appropriate use criteria for amyloid PET imaging: dementia experts, mild cognitive impairment, and education. *J Nucl Med.* 2013;54(7):1011–1013.

Klunk WE, Engler H, Nordberg A, et al. Imaging brain amyloid in Alzheimer's disease with Pittsburgh Compound-B. *Ann Neurol.* 2004;55(3):306–319.

Case 100

PET/CT—RETROPERITONEAL FIBROSIS

1. c
2. d
3. d
4. c

Discussion

This is a case of idiopathic retroperitoneal fibrosis (RF). The etiology is unknown but is thought to be immune mediated. The hallmark imaging finding is that of confluent soft tissue that encases the adjacent vascular structures and, in many cases, the adjacent ureters, which may lead to hydronephrosis and impaired renal function. The underlying pathophysiology is fibrosis. Although most cases are idiopathic, RF may be related to the presence of a malignancy. Other possible causes for secondary RF include medications, infections, surgery, and radiation and immunoglobulin G4–related disease. RF may be FDG avid and therefore may serve as a tool to assess treatment response. Several published reports have documented resolution or decreased FDG avidity after therapy. These masses tend to be enhanced on CT and MRI. The next step in management of this patient is biopsy because other malignancies, such as lymphoma, may have a similar appearance. The treatment generally consists of immunosuppressive therapy and possibly tamoxifen if the patient is unable to receive glucocorticoids. If the ureters are involved, surgery may be considered for decompression and tissue diagnosis, if warranted.

REFERENCES

Jansen I, Hendriksz TR, Han SH, Huiskes AWLC, Van Bommel EFH. 18 F-fluorodeoxyglucose position emission tomography (FDG-PET) for monitoring disease activity and treatment response in idiopathic retroperitoneal fibrosis. *Eur J Intern Med*. 2010;21(3):216–221.

Okuda H, Yamamoto Y, Mitamura K, Norikane T, Nishiyama Y. F-18 FDG PET/CT to monitor disease in patients with IgG4-related disease before and after therapy. *J Nucl Med*. 2017;58(suppl 1):592.

Case 101

CARDIAC AMYLOID

1. b
2. c
3. b
4. c

Discussion

Cardiac amyloidosis may result in restrictive cardiomyopathy, arrhythmias, and/or heart failure. Clinical diagnosis is difficult because symptoms and physical examination findings may mirror other etiologies that may result in heart failure. The gold standard for diagnosis is endocardial biopsy. This is an invasive procedure that is only performed in highly specialized medical centers. Therein lies the need for noninvasive methods for diagnosis and for determination of extent of disease as well as response to therapy. There are two major systemic subtypes: light chain amyloidosis (AL) and transthyretin amyloidosis (ATTR).

Technetium-99m pyrophosphate (Tc-99M PYP) has been utilized for the diagnosis of cardiac amyloidosis. It identifies ATTR. Patients are injected with 15 to 20 mCi of radiopharmaceutical. Approximately an hour after injection, planar and single photon-emission computed tomography (SPECT) images of the chest are obtained. Any uptake within the myocardium is indicative of ATTR. Histologic findings of cardiac amyloidosis are characterized by extracellular fibrillary deposition.

Bone-seeking radiopharmaceuticals have also been shown to bind to myocardium involved in amyloidosis. This is thought to be related to extracellular calcium deposition.

REFERENCES

Bokhari S, Castaño A, Pozniakoff T, Deslisle S, Latif F, Maurer MS. 99m Tc-pyrophosphate scintigraphy for differentiating light-chain cardiac amyloidosis from the transthyretin-related familial and senile cardiac amyloidoses. *Circ Cardiovasc Imaging.* 2013;6(2):195–201.

Ray S, Aahad K, Hussaini S, et al. The increasing burden of amyloidosis from apex to base: new insights from technetium-99m pyrophosphate imaging. *J Am Coll Cardiol.* 2017;69(suppl 11):1521.

Case 102

INDIUM-111 LEUKOCYTES—COLON UPTAKE—COLITIS

1. a
2. b
3. d
4. c

Discussion

This patient was referred for an indium-111 (In-111) leukocyte scan for mild unexplained leukocytosis. There was abnormal uptake in the proximal colon. On a subsequent CT scan, the patient was found to have wall thickening compatible with colitis.

In-111 white blood cell (WBC) scan has normal physiologic uptake in bone marrow, the liver, and the spleen, with splenic uptake normally being greater than liver uptake. Because there is no physiologic intra-abdominal clearance, the In-111 WBC scan is particularly useful for detecting suspected intra-abdominal infection. The Tc-99m hexamethylpropyleneamine oxime (HMPAO)–labeled leukocyte scan shows physiologic urinary and biliary clearance both in the abdomen and in the pelvis.

On day 1 of the scan, blood is drawn from the patient, and labeling of the WBCs occurs over 2 to 3 hours, often at an outside radiopharmacy. The labeled In-111 WBCs are then injected into the patient. If multiple patients are processed the same day, special care must be taken to label each vial/step with patient identifiers to ensure that the patient receives his or her own WBCs during injection. The final preparation will contain radiolabeled granulocytes, lymphocytes, and monocytes. In contrast, Tc-99m HMPAO only radiolabels neutrophils.

Approximately 24 hours later, whole-body planar imaging is performed. If inflammatory bowel disease is suspected, an earlier imaging time point at 4 hours should be considered, because the inflamed mucosal cells slough and uptake seen at 24 hours may not reflect the original site of inflammation.

REFERENCES

Saverymuttu SH, Peters AM, Hodgson H, Chadwick VS, Lavender JP. Indium-111 autologous leucocyte scanning: comparison with radiology for imaging the colon in inflammatory bowel disease. *Br Med J (Clin Res Ed)*. 1982;285(6337):255–257.

Stein DT, Gray GM, Gregory PB, Anderson M, Goodwin DA, Mcdougall LR. Location and activity of ulcerative and Crohn's colitis by indium 111 leukocyte scan. *Gastroenterology*. 1983;84(2):388–393.

Case 103

FRONTOTEMPORAL DEMENTIA (FTD)

1. a
2. b
3. a
4. a

Discussion

This is a fluorine-18 fluorodeoxyglucose positron-emission/computed tomography (F-18 FDG PET/CT) scan of the brain in a patient with altered cognition. The images demonstrated significant hypometabolism in the frontal lobe. Pick's disease is a neurodegenerative disease that causes altered cognition and personality changes. Clinical complaints include memory loss, confusion, and apathy. Clinical deterioration may extend over months or years. In some cases, it is difficult to ascertain whether a patient is suffering from Alzheimer's disease or frontotemporal dementia (FTD). Pick's disease falls under the category of FTD. Molecular imaging studies may be performed to assist with diagnosis. These may be performed with agents such as Tc-99m HMPAO or ethyl cysteinate dimer (EDC; a measure of perfusion) or F-18 FDG (a measure of metabolic activity). Alzheimer's disease is characterized by decreased perfusion (metabolism) in the posterior (parietal and temporal) cortices, whereas Pick's disease demonstrates decreased perfusion (metabolism) in the frontal lobes and anterior temporal lobes.

REFERENCES

Mendez MF, Selwood A, Mastri AR, Frey W. Pick's disease versus Alzheimer's disease a comparison of clinical characteristics. *Neurology*. 1993;43(2):289.

Kamo H, McGeer PL, Harrop R, et al. Positron emission tomography and histopathology in Pick's disease. *Neurology*. 1987;37(3):439.

Case 104

SCINTIMAMMOGRAPHY—TC-99M SESTAMIBI—BREAST CANCER

1. b
2. b
3. d
4. c

Discussion

This case shows a focus of uptake in the left breast at the 3 o'clock position. This corresponded to a 1-cm spiculated lesion on a dedicated mammogram (not pictured). This lesion was biopsied and found to represent invasive ductal carcinoma.

Mammography is the mainstay imaging modality for breast cancer screening. The reported sensitivity for conventional mammography is 75% to 95%. However, low specificity results in high number of benign biopsy results. Tomosynthesis is thought to have improved the specificity of screening. In particular, screening mammography is difficult to perform in women with dense breasts, breast implants, or a history of prior surgery. Women with fatty breasts do not present the same difficulties in mammographic screening. Scintigraphic techniques utilize Tc-99m sestamibi. Sestamibi binds to mitochondria within the cells. It is not affected by density of breasts or surgery. Radiotracer uptake does not occur only in the setting of breast cancer. False-positive results may be seen in the setting of fibroadenoma and fibrocystic changes. Small lesions (<1 cm) may cause a false-negative result. NPO (nothing by mouth) status is not required before study. Insulin administration has no effect on study quality. It is recommended that the study be delayed if core biopsy or excisional biopsy has been performed within 4 to 6 weeks *or* a cyst aspiration or fine-needle aspiration within 2 weeks. Dedicated breast imaging gamma cameras that have allowed for reduction in radiation dose and improved spatial resolution have been developed.

REFERENCES

Fenlon HM, Phelan NC, O'Sullivan P, Tierney S, Gorey T, Ennis JT. Benign versus malignant breast disease: comparison of contrast-enhanced MR imaging and Tc-99m tetrofosmin scintimammography. *Radiology*. 1997;205(1):214–220.

Goldsmith SJ, Parsons W, Guiberteau MJ, et al. SNM practice guideline for breast scintigraphy with breast-specific γ-cameras 1.0. *J Nucl Med Technol*. 2010;38(4):219–224.

Khalkhali I, Cutrone JA, Mena IG, et al. Scintimammography: the complementary role of Tc-99m sestamibi prone breast imaging for the diagnosis of breast carcinoma. *Radiology*. 1995;196(2):421–442.

Case 105

F-18 FDG PET—ELASTOFIBROMA DORSI

1. a
2. d
3. a
4. c

Discussion

This case demonstrates an FDG-avid soft tissue lesion at the inferior aspect of the right scapula. Elastofibroma dorsi is a benign, ill-defined fibroelastic pseudotumor affecting elderly patients and occurring mainly in a subscapular location. The CT shows lenticular areas of soft tissue attenuation similar to that of muscle with linear areas of interspersed fat attenuation. Patients may be asymptomatic or may have pain or a sensation of clicking. Findings are most commonly seen in older women, and up to 60% are bilateral. Low-grade uptake within the lesions has been documented on F-18 FDG PET/CT studies.

REFERENCES

Ochsner JE, Sewall SA, Brooks GN, Agni R. Elastofibroma dorsi. *Radiographics*. 2006;26(6):1873–1876.

Patrikeos A, Breidahl W, Robins P. F-18 FDG uptake associated with Elastofibroma dorsi. *Clin Nucl Med*. 2005;30(9):617–618.

Case 106

BONE SCAN—POLYOSTOTIC FIBROUS DYSPLASIA

1. a
2. b
3. a
4. d

Discussion

This is a bone scan of a patient who presented with bone pain. The scan demonstrates multiple foci of abnormal radiotracer uptake in the bony structures. The left femur shows a classic "shepherd's crook" deformity, which is characteristic of fibrous dysplasia.

Fibrous dysplasia is a benign bony disorder characterized by abnormal proliferation of fibroblasts resulting in fibrous tissue replacing normal bone. Because of this, bone becomes weak and is prone to injuries, such as fracture. This condition may be monostotic or polyostotic. It is most frequently diagnosed in younger (<20 years of age) patients. Most lesions demonstrate radiotracer uptake above that of background bone. If a lesion involves the craniofacial structures, it may lead to hearing or vision loss, as well as facial deformities. In the setting of polyostotic disease, a third of patients will have café au lait spots. These skin lesions have an irregular margin in contrast to café au lait spots that tend to have smooth margins, seen in the setting of neurofibromatosis. Precocious puberty may occur in up to 30% of women with polyostotic disease, and this is referred to as *McCune-Albright syndrome*. Bone scintigraphy is useful for evaluating whether this is a mono- or polyostotic disease, as well as for the assessment of lesion extent. No curative treatment is available, and the mainstay of treatment is palliative. Bisphosphonates have been used for the treatment of bone pain. Ollier's and Maffucci's syndromes are associated with enchondromas of the bone, whereas Zollinger-Ellison syndrome is associated with gastrinomas.

REFERENCES

Chapurlat RD, Orcel P. Fibrous dysplasia of bone and McCune–Albright syndrome. *Best Pract Res Clin Rheumatol*. 2008;22(1):55–69.
DiCaprio MR, Enneking WF. Fibrous dysplasia: pathophysiology, evaluation, and treatment. *JBJS*. 2005;87(8):1848–1864.

Case 107

F-18 FDG PET—CRANIOPHARYNGIOMA

1. b
2. c
3. c
4. a

Discussion

The F-18 FDG PET/CT brain images demonstrate reduced focal uptake (photopenic defect) in the suprasellar region (Image A). This case illustrates the importance of identifying abnormal areas of increased or absent FDG avidity. This lesion was incidentally discovered on F-18 FDG PET/CT performed as a workup for a systemic malignancy unrelated to the presence of craniopharyngioma. The CT component clearly demonstrated a cystic lesion in the suprasellar region associated with areas if calcification on CT (Image B), most compatible with a craniopharyngioma. The patient went on to have magnetic resonance imaging (MRI) of the brain (Image C), which demonstrated a mixed cystic solid lesion centered at the suprasellar cistern. Histopathology after resection confirmed the diagnosis.

Craniopharyngiomas are benign World Health Organization grade I tumors. They represent approximately 1% to 5% of primary brain tumors. The distribution of patients diagnosed with craniopharyngiomas is bimodal, occurring in the early teens and then again after age 50 years. Patients may present with headaches, visual disturbances, and/or hormonal imbalances. These lesions can also be discovered incidentally. Almost all of these lesions involve both the sellar and suprasellar compartments and, when large enough, may extend to the optic chiasm or adjacent lobes. It is important to note, however, that ectopic lesions have been described in the literature. Treatment usually involves surgical resection with possible focal radiotherapy, if indicated. The differential diagnosis includes Rathke's cleft cyst, which would also be photopenic.

REFERENCES

Chapurlat RD, Orcel P. Fibrous dysplasia of bone and McCune–Albright syndrome. *Best Pract Res Clin Rheumatol.* 2008;22(1):55–69.

Ryu SI, Tafti BA, Skirboll SL. Pituitary adenomas can appear as hypermetabolic lesions in 18F-FDG PET imaging. *J Neuroimaging.* 2010;20(4):393–396.

Case 108

MIBG—PHEOCHROMOCYTOMA/PARAGANGLIOMA— METASTATIC PHEOCHROMOCYTOMA

1. b
2. c
3. c
4. a

Discussion

This is a case of metastatic pheochromocytoma/paraganglioma. These tumors that arise from the neural crest tissues are rare. Patients may present with symptoms related to catecholamine excess, including hypertension, headache, and palpitations. There is usually evidence of elevated serum and urinary catecholamines. Symptoms are classically paroxysmal.

This iodine-123 metaiodobenzylguanidine (I-123 MIBG) scan demonstrates multiple abnormal foci of increased radiotracer uptake, compatible with metastatic disease.

The radiotracer binds to norepinephrine receptors. Characteristics that predict aggressive behavior at diagnosis (assuming no metastasis at diagnosis) include large size of the primary lesion, primary lesion outside the adrenal gland (paraganglioma), and associated enzymatic defects, including succinyl dehydrogenase enzyme defect. Metastatic disease may be treated with I-131 MIBG intravenous therapy. Lu-177 PSMA may be indicated for the treatment of prostate cancer, and yttrium-90 (Y-90) microspheres have been used for primary and metastatic liver lesions.

REFERENCES

Greenblatt DY, Shenker Y, Chen H. The utility of metaiodobenzylguanidine (MIBG) scintigraphy in patients with pheochromocytoma. *Ann Surg Oncol.* 2008;15(3):900–905.

Meyer-Rochow GY, Schembri GP, Benn DE, et al. The utility of metaiodobenzylguanidine single photon emission computed tomography/computed tomography (MIBG SPECT/CT) for the diagnosis of pheochromocytoma. *Ann Surg Oncol.* 2010;17(2):392–400.

Case 109

I-123 WHOLE BODY SCAN AND F-18 FDG PET/CT— PAPILLARY THYROID CANCER

1. a
2. b
3. c
4. c

Discussion

Papillary thyroid cancer (PTC) is the most common primary malignancy of the thyroid gland. PTC is typically iodine avid and can be imaged with I-123 and treated with I-131. If, however, PTC is not iodine avid on imaging, the disease cannot be treated with I-131. Patients who present with PTC initially undergo thyroid resection and perhaps I-131 therapy, depending on the stage and histology of the tumor. Follow-up may consist of I-123 imaging 1 year after surgery and, with positive results, I-131 therapy. If the workup at 1 year shows negative results, serum thyroglobulin levels are then routinely monitored for recurrent disease.

Should serum thyroglobulin levels rise, an I-123 whole-body scan is performed to assess for recurrent disease. FDG PET/CT plays a valuable role in the post-thyroidectomy workup of patients who have elevated thyroglobulin levels and a negative I-123 scan result. As thyroid cancer cells dedifferentiate, correlating with higher-grade disease, their radioiodine uptake usually decreases, and their glucose metabolism generally increases. FDG PET/CT is not indicated in the assessment of lower-grade disease because of low sensitivity. If nodal disease is identified on FDG PET, surgical excision is indicated. F-18 fluciclovine is used to evaluate prostate cancer. I-131 whole body imaging would not be expected to add any value following a negative I-123 scan.

REFERENCES

Schlüter B, Bohuslavizki KH, Beyer W, Plotkin M, Buchert R, Clausen M. Impact of FDG PET on patients with differentiated thyroid cancer who present with elevated thyroglobulin and negative 131I scan. *J Nucl Med*. 2001;42(1):71–76.

Shammas A, Degirmenci B, Mountz JM, et al. 18F-FDG PET/CT in patients with suspected recurrent or metastatic well-differentiated thyroid cancer. *J Nucl Med*. 2007;48(2):221–226.

Case 110

F-18 FDG PET—SODIUM FLUORIDE (NAF)

1. b
2. b
3. c
4. b

Discussion

F-18 NaF received the U.S. Food and Drug Administration (FDA) approval in 1972 for use in the evaluation of bone metastases. However, at that time, imaging equipment was not sufficient to adequately depict high-energy photons. Hence, Tc-99m methyl diphosphonate (MDP) has remained for decades the mainstay in the scintigraphic evaluation of bone metastases. More recently, with the increased availability of PET/CT scanners, there has been a resurgence of interest in exploring the role of F-18 NaF PET/CT in the evaluation of bone metastases. F-18 NaF is more sensitive for detection of bone metastases compared with the Tc-99m MDP bone scan, likely because of the increased bone uptake of NaF as well as the increased spatial resolution of PET/CT. The CT component gives the study high specificity.

Sensitivity is the true-positive rate, and specificity is the true-negative rate. No special preparation is needed before imaging. Before initiation of imaging, patients should be encouraged to void the bladder. The bladder receives the highest radiation dose, and therefore patients should be encouraged to drink fluids and urinate frequently after the examination. Radiotracer uptake is related to increased bone turnover. It is important to note that areas of degenerative change, as well as benign bone processes, such as fibrous dysplasia, will demonstrate increased radiotracer uptake. Standardized uptake value (SUV) measurements cannot differentiate between benign and malignant etiologies.

REFERENCES

Hetzel M, Arslandemir C, König HH, et al. F-18 NaF PET for detection of bone metastases in lung cancer: accuracy, cost-effectiveness, and impact on patient management. *J Bone Miner Res.* 2003;18(12): 2206–2214.

Iagaru A, Mittra E, Dick DW, Gambhir SS. Prospective evaluation of 99mTc MDP scintigraphy, 18F NaF PET/CT, and 18F FDG PET/CT for detection of skeletal metastases. *Mol Imaging Biol.* 2012;14(2):252–259.

Case 111

F-18 FDG PET—CARDIAC SARCOID

1. a
2. b
3. a
4. c

Discussion

Sarcoidosis, a relatively uncommon systemic granulomatous disease of unknown etiology, may affect multiple organ systems. Sarcoidosis frequently involves the mediastinal and hilar nodes, resulting in lymph node enlargement. Sarcoid manifestations in the lungs vary, depending on the patient's age and the stage of the disease. Findings may be described as nodular opacities, air space opacities, and possibly fibrosis and bronchiectasis. Cardiac involvement may occur in one out of four patients with sarcoidosis. Sarcoid involvement of the myocardium may result in scarring/fibrosis. The clinical manifestations of cardiac sarcoidosis range from subclinical disease to arrhythmias and conduction defects to cardiac arrest. Accurate diagnosis of cardiac sarcoid is difficult. Endomyocardial biopsy of the myocardium is invasive and has low sensitivity, in part because of sampling error. In light of this, there has been increased interest in utilizing imaging techniques, such as MRI and PET/CT, to assess for underlying cardiac sarcoidosis.

F-18 FDG uptake in cardiac sarcoidosis is thought to be related to uptake in increased macrophage activity at the site of disease. Although the myocardium primarily gains energy from fatty acid metabolism, the normal myocardium may also metabolize glucose and hence demonstrate increased uptake. This uptake may be diffuse or patchy and may be seen even in patients who are NPO. Hence, myocardial suppression of glucose uptake must be performed. Two main methods have been considered: prolonged fasting (some studies suggesting >18 hours) and a high-fat/high-protein/low-carbohydrate diet before imaging. A combination of the two methods may also be performed. When evaluating for cardiac sarcoidosis, a resting cardiac perfusion PET/CT scan with either NH-13 ammonia or rubidium-82 is performed, and this is followed by F-18 FDG scan. The classic finding of cardiac sarcoidosis is a mismatched pattern with decreased perfusion at the site of increased F-18 FDG uptake, as seen in this case (best seen on polar maps). Focal uptake related to sarcoidosis tends to occur at the base of the septum or lateral wall, although uptake may occur anywhere in the myocardium in a diffuse or focal distribution.

REFERENCES

Harisankar, NC, et al. Utility of high fat and low carbohydrate diet in suppressing myocardial FDG uptake. *J Nucl Cardiol*. 2011;18(5):926.

Schatka I, Bengel FM. Advanced imaging of cardiac sarcoidosis. *J Nucl Med*. 2014;55(1):99–106.

Schindler Thomas H, Solnes LS. Role of PET/CT for the identification of cardiac sarcoid disease. *Ann Nucl Cardiol*. 2015;1(1):79–86.

Case 112

F-18 FDG PET—EWING'S SARCOMA

1. b
2. b
3. b
4. a

Discussion

This is a case of Ewing's sarcoma involving the left scapula. Ewing's sarcoma is the second most common malignant osseous tumor in children and young adults. These tumors tend to be ill-defined osseous lesions arising from an intramedullary location and extending into adjacent soft tissues. The most common complaint is localized pain. These permeative, ill-defined lesions occur most commonly in the diaphysis or metadiaphysis of long bones, although they may also be seen at other sites. This is typically a monostotic disease. These lesions are three-phase positive on bone scans. MRI with contrast is the ideal imaging technique for the evaluation of the extent of the primary lesion and for surgical planning. Metastatic disease tends to involve bones or lungs. Studies show that F-18 FDG PET has greater sensitivity and specificity for detecting osseous metastases compared with bone scintigraphy. The degree of FDG uptake is thought to correlate with tumor grade.

REFERENCES

Charest M, Hickeson M, Lisbona R, Novales-Diaz JA, Derbekyan V, Turcotte RE. FDG PET/CT imaging in primary osseous and soft tissue sarcomas: a retrospective review of 212 cases. *Eur J Nucl Med Mol Imaging*. 2009;35(12):1944.

Franzius C, Sciuk J, Daldrup-Link HE, Jürgens H, Schober O. FDG-PET for detection of osseous metastases from malignant primary bone tumours: comparison with bone scintigraphy. *Eur J Nucl Med*. 2000;27(9):1305–1311.

Case 113

TERTIARY HYPERPARATHYROIDISM

1. d
2. b
3. b
4. a

Discussion

This Tc-99m sestamibi scan of the parathyroid glands demonstrates three foci of increased radiotracer uptake in the neck. The patient had long-standing chronic renal failure and now has tertiary hyperparathyroidism. Patients with chronic renal failure initially have secondary hyperparathyroidism with hypocalcemia and increased parathyroid hormone (PTH) levels, causing parathyroid hyperplasia, but the serum calcium level remains low. The poor kidney function results in decreased active vitamin D, and this causes poor absorption of calcium from the gastrointestinal tract and reabsorption from the kidneys, thus causing hypocalcemia and increased PTH. The majority of patients with secondary hyperparathyroidism can be effectively treated with calcitriol (metabolite of vitamin D). However, in some patients, this is ineffective, and one or more glands become autonomous, causing tertiary hyperparathyroidism with elevated calcium levels and PTH. In these cases, surgery is required. The parathyroid scan can localize the offending gland(s) for the surgeon. SPECT/CT can be helpful for better localization.

REFERENCES

Eslamy HK, Ziessman HA. Parathyroid scintigraphy in patients with primary hyperparathyroidism: 99mTc sestamibi SPECT and SPECT/CT. *Radiographics*. 2008;28(5):1461–1476.

Loftus KA, Anderson S, Mulloy AL, Terris DJ. Value of sestamibi scans in tertiary hyperparathyroidism. *The Laryngoscope*. 2007;117(12):2135–2138.

Case 114

F-18 FDG PET—CORTICAL DYSPLASIA

1. a
2. d
3. a
4. d

Discussion

The F-18 FDG PET/CT of the brain demonstrates focal decreased uptake in the left frontal region. There are many possible possible causes, including infarcts, low-grade tumors, and seizure foci (interictal), as well as prior insults, such as infarcts or interventions. An ictal seizure focus would have increased uptake. Clinical history is critical when interpreting these scans. This patient had a history of complex partial seizures. MRI of the brain was subsequently performed; Image B demonstrates cortical dysplasia in the region of the metabolic defect. Physiologic cortical activity should never be photopenic.

Cortical dysplasia is a developmental anomaly resulting from failed migration of neurons. MRI is optimal for diagnosis. Imaging features on MRI include cortical thickening, increased fluid-attenuated inversion recovery (FLAIR) or T2 signal, abnormal sulcal/gyral pattern, and blurring of the gray–white junction. Cortical dysplasia can cause seizures. The FDG scan can not only help with differential diagnosis but also confirm other clinical information regarding the site of seizure, for example, from electroencephalography (EEG).

REFERENCES

Kim SK, Na DG, Byun HS, et al. Focal cortical dysplasia: comparison of MRI and FDG-PET. *J Comput Assist Tomogr*. 2000;24(2): 296–302.

Spencer SS. The relative contributions of MRI, SPECT, and PET imaging in epilepsy. *Epilepsia*. 1994;35(s6):S72–S89.

Case 115

TC-99M HIDA—FOCAL NODULAR HYPERPLASIA (FNH)

1. c
2. b
3. c
4. a

Discussion

Hepatobiliary iminodiacetic acid (HIDA) radiopharmaceuticals are taken up by hepatocytes and excreted into the biliary system without conjugation. This HIDA study shows a focus of increased radiotracer uptake at the inferior tip of the right lobe of the liver; the increased uptake becomes more apparent as the radiotracer is excreted from the liver. This focus has an appearance of a rounded lesion, which corresponds to an ovoid hepatic mass that is relatively isointense to the adjacent liver parenchyma on the coronal MRI (fast imaging employing steady-state acquisition [FIESTA]).

Focal nodular hyperplasia (FNH) is the second most common benign tumor of the liver. Eighty to 95% of FNH cases are found in women, most commonly in their third or fourth decade of life. FNH is a hamartomatous mass—a proliferation of normal non-neoplastic hepatocytes that are abnormally arranged. On a Tc-99m HIDA scan, FNH typically shows increased flow, increased radiotracer uptake, and delayed clearance of tracer. Delayed clearance is thought to be related to the abnormal bile canaliculi that do not communicate with the normal biliary system. Findings in the above case are consistent with an FNH. FNH may also be identified on Tc-99m SC scans. Because these lesions contain functioning Kupffer's cells, the radiopharmaceutical will accumulate in these lesions. Approximately two-thirds of these will show uptake similar or above that of adjacent normal liver. The remainder will be relatively photopenic.

FNH has no malignant potential, and thus management is typically conservative. Surgery is considered in atypical cases when differentiation from hepatic adenoma or other tumors is difficult or if the patient is symptomatic because of lesion size.

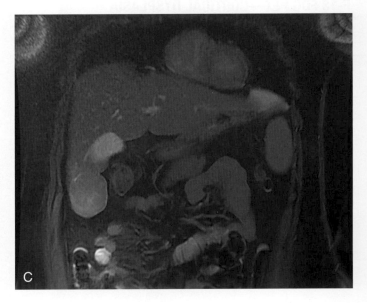

Estrogen may be associated with the growth of FNH, although this notion is somewhat controversial, and discontinuation of oral contraceptives may be considered.

Hemangioma, which does not contain functioning hepatocytes, would be photopenic on the HIDA study. Despite being composed of hepatocytes, hepatic adenomas do not show radiotracer uptake, which is thought to result from the absence of bile ducts in the adenoma.

REFERENCE

Biersack HJ, Thelen M, Torres JF, Lackner K, Winkler CG. Focal nodular hyperplasia of the liver as established by 99mTc sulfur colloid and HIDA scintigraphy. *Radiology*. 1980;137(1):187–190.

Case 116

F-18 FDG PET—ENDOCARDITIS

1. a
2. a
3. b
4. a

Discussion

This is a case of endocarditis identified on an F-18 FDG PET/CT. Circumferential uptake is seen in the region of the aortic valve. The workup of endocarditis includes blood cultures as well as a transesophageal echocardiography (TEE). An In-111 WBC SPECT/CT may also be considered as an alternative to FDG PET for the evaluation of endocarditis. F-18 FDG PET cannot be used in isolation for making the diagnosis of endocarditis. However, as improvements in patient preparation are made and technical advances in instrumentation evolve, FDG PET/CT may play a greater role in the evaluation for endocarditis.

Whole-body FDG PET/CT likely plays a greater role in evaluating for a source of infection. Physiologic activity is not generally seen in the region of the aortic valve. Myocardial infarction may initially demonstrate increased tracer activity because of inflammation. This activity is generally confined to the myocardium in the vascular distribution of an infarction.

REFERENCES

Fagman E, van Essen M, Lindqvist JF, Snygg-Martin U, Bech-Hanssen O, Svensson G. 18F-FDG PET/CT in the diagnosis of prosthetic valve endocarditis. *Int J Cardiovasc Imaging*. 2016;32(4):679–686.

Kouijzer IJ, Vos FJ, Janssen MJ, van Dijk AP, Oyen WJ, Bleeker-Rovers CP. The value of 18F-FDG PET/CT in diagnosing infectious endocarditis. *Eur J Nucl Med Mol Imaging*. 2013;40(7):1102–1107.

Case 117

PET/CT PLEXIFORM NEUROFIBROMAS IN NF1

1. c
2. b
3. c
4. d

Discussion

Neurofibromatosis type 1 (NF1) is a relatively common autosomal dominant disease. Patients may develop cutaneous and plexiform neurofibromas, café au lait spots, Lisch's nodules, optic gliomas, and bone dysplasias. Plexiform neurofibromas may degenerate into malignant nerve sheath tumors. Both lesions may manifest with pain, increasing size, and new neurologic symptoms, making clinical examination for differentiation difficult. This case demonstrates multiple plexiform neurofibromas in the lower extremity as well as in the left axilla. Cross-sectional imaging cannot reliably differentiate between benign and malignant forms. Most malignant nerve sheath tumors arise from plexiform neurofibromas. The lifetime risk of transformation is about 10%. Molecular imaging with F-18 FDG PET/CT has been employed to evaluate for transformation. The general idea being that as these lesions transform, they become more metabolically active.

REFERENCES

Chirindel A, Chaudhry M, Blakeley JO, Wahl R. 18F-FDG PET/CT qualitative and quantitative evaluation in neurofibromatosis type 1 patients for detection of malignant transformation: comparison of early to delayed imaging with and without liver activity normalization. *J Nucl Med*. 2015;56(3):379–385.

Nguyen R, Jett K, Harris GJ, Cai W, Friedman JM, Mautner VF. Benign whole body tumor volume is a risk factor for malignant peripheral nerve sheath tumors in neurofibromatosis type 1. *J Neurooncol*. 2014;116(2):307–313.

Case 118

PET/CT—GA-68 DOTA-TATE

1. c
2. a
3. c
4. c

Discussion

This is a gallium-68 (Ga-68) DOTA-TATE scan (Image A) performed for the evaluation of a neuroendocrine tumor (NET). This case demonstrates focal abnormal signal in the region of the pancreas, corresponding to an NET as seen on dedicated CT images (Images B and C). In addition, there is an abnormal focus of radiotracer uptake in the left posterior fossa, which was an incidentally detected meningioma (Images D and E). Meningiomas express somatostatin receptors.

Ga-68 DOTA-TATE was approved by the FDA in 2016. Neuroendocrine tumors are uncommon tumors, traditionally evaluated with conventional anatomic imaging (CT and MRI) and In 111-pentetreotide (Octreoscan). Similar to Octreoscan, Ga-68 DOTA-TATE targets somatostatin receptors. The radiopharmaceutical almost exclusively targets somatostatin receptor II and has a much greater affinity for the receptor compared with Octreoscan. The normal biodistribution includes the pituitary gland, thyroid gland, adrenals, kidneys, pancreas, prostate, liver, and salivary glands. In contrast to FDG PET/CT, there is no physiologic uptake in the cerebrum. There are some potential pitfalls one must be aware of. These include normal focal uptake in the uncinate process of the pancreas as well as in inflammatory lymph nodes. Also, as these tumors dedifferentiate, they lose their somatostatin receptor expression and therefore may produce a false-negative result. Compared with Octreoscan, Ga-68 DOTA-TATE detects more lesions and may lead to changes in management in up to 50% of cases.

REFERENCES

Hofman MS, Kong G, Neels OC, Eu P, Hong E, Hicks RJ. High management impact of Ga-68 DOTATATE (GaTate) PET/CT for imaging neuroendocrine and other somatostatin expressing tumours. *J Med Imaging Radiat Oncol*. 2012;56(1):40–47.

Case 119

F-18 FDG PET—PROSTATE ABSCESS

1. c
2. b
3. a
4. a

Discussion

Images demonstrate intensely avid, hypodense lesions within an enlarged prostate gland. Prostate abscesses are a rare complication of prostatitis. This is a serious condition that may be life threatening. Common symptoms include fever, dysuria, suprapubic pain, and tenderness in the region of the prostate. CT findings include an enlarged prostate with rim-enhancing loculated or multiloculated fluid collections, as noted in this case. Prompt diagnosis is paramount in these patients. Prostate adenocarcinoma is not typically intensely hypermetabolic on FDG PET/CT and would not typically present with multiple fluid collections.

REFERENCES

Thornhill Beverly A, et al. Prostatic abscess: CT and sonographic findings. *Am J Roentgenol.* 1987;148(5):899–900.

Case 120

F-18 FDG PET—METASTATIC PULMONARY CALCIFICATIONS

1. c
2. c
3. d
4. a

Discussion

This case is an example of metastatic pulmonary calcification (MPC). The images show hypermetabolic activity associated with "fluffy" ground-glass nodular densities in the lung apices. The bandlike uptake in the lower neck is physiologic muscle uptake.

Metastatic pulmonary calcification is a well-recognized complication of end-stage renal disease secondary to abnormal calcium metabolism. The etiology of metastatic pulmonary calcification is presumably related to the balance of serum calcium, phosphate, and vitamin D. Reported risk factors include hypercalcemia, hyperphosphatemia, and elevated plasma calcium–phosphate product. Calcium deposition in normal lung parenchyma at the apices is thought to be caused by a more alkaline environment resulting from the increased ventilation/perfusion ratio at the apices.

The most common presentation is seen in patients on hemodialysis for chronic renal failure with secondary hyperparathyroidism. Other conditions in which this finding may be observed include widespread bone destruction from metastases or multiple myeloma (as in this case), sarcoidosis, and hypervitaminosis D. Treatment of this condition is primarily symptomatic, which includes lowering of calcium–phosphate products in the body with use of phosphate binders.

The associated activity on FDG PET is presumably secondary to associated inflammatory changes. MPC may be incidentally noted on bone scans as increased uptake of the radiotracer within the lungs and the stomach.

REFERENCES

Hartman TE, Müller NL, Primack SL, et al. Metastatic pulmonary calcification in patients with hypercalcemia: findings on chest radiographs and CT scans. *Am J Roentgenol.* 1994;162(4):799–802.

Case 121

HIDA HEPATOBRONCHIAL FISTULA

1. a
2. a
3. c
4. a

Discussion

This patient presented with bilious vomiting after resection of hepatic metastasis from colon cancer. The HIDA scan demonstrated abnormal Tc-99m mebrofenin radiotracer transiting from the biliary tree to the bronchial tree. Bronchobiliary fistulas are very rare complications usually related to hepatic or subdiaphragmatic abscesses. Other possible causes include hepatic tumors or prior interventions, such as surgery or radiofrequency embolization. Patients may present with cough and biliptysis (bile in cough) as well as right upper quadrant pain and fever. Diagnosis may be accomplished with MRI or hepatobiliary scanning. Treatments often involve surgery or endoscopic intervention.

REFERENCES

Liao Guan-Qun, et al. Management of acquired bronchobiliary fistula: a systematic literature review of 68 cases published in 30 years. *World J Gastroenterol*. 2011;17(33):3842.

Mandal Ajay, Sen Sanjay, Baig Sarfaraz Jalil. Bronchobiliary fistula. *J Minim Access Surg*. 2008;4(4):111.

Case 122

F-18 FDG PET—FAT NECROSIS

1. c
2. b
3. a
4. d

Discussion

Intra-abdominal fat may undergo necrosis, causing inflammation and abdominal pain, mimicking an acute abdomen in some patients. Some of the common forms of fat necrosis in the abdomen caused by vascular compromise include omental infarction and epiploic appendagitis. Trauma and pancreatitis may also cause localized fat necrosis.

The general appearance of fat necrosis on CT (as seen in this case) is a region of central fat surrounded by a rim of soft tissue attenuation and variable adjacent soft tissue stranding and infiltration.

In epiploic appendagitis, the epiploic appendages, which are small outpouchings of visceral peritoneum that contain fat and small blood vessels arising from the serosal surface adjacent to the tenia coli in the colon, infarct from torsion or occlusion of the central vessel. Similarly, omental fat may infarct in areas of tenuous blood supply or as a result of torsion. Omental infarction more commonly occurs in the right abdomen but may occur in the left abdomen as well (as in this case). Fat necrosis is FDG avid on PET/CT, reflecting the inflammatory response. Fat necrosis is a self-limiting process, treated conservatively with pain management. It is important to be aware of this diagnosis so as not to confuse it with malignancy. In this case, the abnormal region of uptake was initially attributed to the colon and assumed to represent malignancy.

REFERENCES

Kamaya A, Federle MP, Desser TS. Imaging manifestations of abdominal fat necrosis and its mimics. *Radiographics*. 2011;31(7):2021–2034.

Case 123

I-123 MIBG—NEUROBLASTOMA

1. a
2. b
3. b
4. c

Discussion

This is an I-123 MIBG scan that demonstrates abnormal radiotracer activity in the region of the left adrenal gland (better visualized on posterior images). In addition, there is focal uptake in the right femur consistent with osseous metastases. Axial CT images demonstrate a large heterogeneous mass in the left adrenal bed associated with calcifications. Findings are consistent with neuroblastoma.

Neuroblastomas arise from the sympathetic nervous system. Most patients are younger than 4 years of age at diagnosis.

The most common site of primary disease is the retroperitoneal region, which includes the adrenal glands and the retroperitoneal sympathetic chain. The second most common primary site is the thoracic sympathetic chain. About half the patients at diagnosis will have metastatic disease. Patients with only local disease have a much better prognosis compared with patients with metastatic disease. Metastatic disease typically involves the lymph nodes, bone/bone marrow, and liver. The standard workup of the neuroblastoma includes an I-123 MIBG scan. MIBG sensitivity for detection is approximately 90% and specificity is 95%. When combined with bone scanning, the highest detection for metastatic disease can be achieved.

REFERENCES

Sharp SE, Shulkin BL, Gelfand MJ, Salisbury S, Furman WL. 123I-MIBG scintigraphy and 18F-FDG PET in neuroblastoma. *J Nucl Med.* 2009;50(8):1237–1243.

Case 124

F-18 FDG PET—ENCEPHALITIS

1. a
2. a
3. a
4. a

Discussion

Increased FLAIR/T2 signal is seen on MRI in bilateral medial temporal lobes of this patient and is associated with F-18 FDG avidity on dedicated PET/CT. Autoimmune encephalitis (AE) is challenging to diagnose because of the heterogeneity of symptoms that are difficult to characterize. Reported symptoms may include seizures, confusion, mental status changes, and behavioral disturbances. Imaging studies may not demonstrate focal abnormalities. When present, MRI findings that suggest the diagnosis include increased FLAIR/T2 signal in the medial temporal lobes. This finding may be unilateral or bilateral. This may or may not be associated with increased FDG avidity in the medial temporal lobes on PET/CT. Imaging findings may extend into areas beyond the medial temporal lobe. AE may be associated with underlying malignancies, although this is not always the case. Some of the more common tumors associated with AE include small cell lung cancer, germ cell tumors, and breast cancers. Nonparaneoplastic AE may be seen in the setting of anti-N-methyl-D-aspartate (anti-NMDA), which is commonly in seen in young woman with a history of teratomas. Antibodies, in general, will affect with surface antigens or intracellular antigens. If symptoms of fever and cognitive changes occur acutely, herpes encephalitis should be considered.

REFERENCES

Solnes LB, Jones KM, Rowe SP, et al. Diagnostic value of ^{18}F-FDG PET/CT versus MRI in the setting of antibody specific autoimmune encephalitis. *J Nucl Med.* 2017;58(8):1307–1313.

Case 125

PET PTLD

1. b
2. c
3. c
4. a

Discussion

This F-18 FDG PET/CT demonstrates a right lower quadrant kidney compatible with history of transplantation as well as large bowel wall thickening associated with increased FDG avidity. This is a case of post-transplant lymphoproliferative disease (PTLD) after renal transplantation. PTLD is the second most common malignancy that occurs after transplantation. PTLD is often associated with Epstein-Barr virus in the setting of immunosuppression. There are several histologic types ranging from benign lymphoid hyperplasia to poorly differentiated lymphoma. Less aggressive histologic lesions may respond to withdrawal of immunosuppression, whereas more aggressive lesions require more invasive measures such as surgery, chemotherapy, and radiation. The incidence of PTLD is thought to be related to the type of transplant as well as specific immunosuppression therapies. PTLD generally occurs within the first year of transplantation or 4 to 5 years after transplantation. Although PTLD may present as nodal disease, extranodal manifestations are more common. The most common site of disease is the abdomen. Tissue sampling is required to determine the histologic grade.

REFERENCES

Camacho JC, Moreno CC, Peter HA, et al. Posttransplantation lymphoproliferative disease: proposed imaging classification. *Radiographics*. 2014;34(7):2025–2038.

Case 126

LYMPHOSCINTIGRAPHY—EPITROCHLEAR SENTINEL LYMPH NODE

1. a
2. c
3. c
4. a

Discussion

This case illustrates the presence of an epitrochlear lymph node on lymphoscintigraphy. When performing lymphoscintigraphy of the upper extremity for melanomas, it is important to be aware of their presence. Epitrochlear lymph nodes are superficial, located in the region of the medial elbow and generally drain the medial hand, third through fifth digits. There may be one to four nodes. It is particularly important to identify these lymph nodes in patients with upper extremity melanoma. The nodes are considered transit/interval sentinel nodes, which may harbor metastases. Lymphoscintigraphy is performed for surgical mapping and preoperative planning. In patients with melanoma, epitrochlear nodes may be the only site of disease. Because lymph node involvement is an important predictor of outcome in melanoma, identification of epitrochlear nodes is paramount.

REFERENCES

Catalano O, Nunziata A, Saturnino PP, Siani A. Epitrochlear lymph nodes: anatomy, clinical aspects, and sonography features. Pictorial essay. *J Ultrasound.* 2010;13(4):168–174.

McMasters KM, Chao C, Wong SL, Wrightson WR, Ross MI, Reintgen DS. Interval sentinel lymph nodes in melanoma. *Arch Surg.* 2002;137(5):543–547.

Case 127

F-18 FDG PET—HAMARTOMA

1. a
2. c
3. b
4. d

Discussion

FDG PET/CT has a role in the evaluation of pulmonary nodules. The 2017 Fleischner's Society guidelines recommend consideration of PET/CT for solid nodules 8 mm or greater in size.

Benign pulmonary hamartomas characteristically contain macroscopic fat. Those that do not contain fat cannot be characterized as benign by imaging alone. These lesions do not tend to demonstrate significantly increased F-18 FDG uptake on PET/CT. Pathologically proven hamartomas have an SUV_{max} range of 0.7 to 2.2. Other lesions that typically show absent or low-grade activity include bronchopulmonary carcinoid tumor, adenocarcinoma in situ, and minimally invasive adenocarcinoma.

The pulmonary lesion in this case, shown above, contains fat and is consistent with the diagnosis of a benign hamartoma.

REFERENCES

MacMahon H, Naidich DP, Goo JM, et al. Guidelines for management of incidental pulmonary nodules detected on CT images: from the Fleischner Society 2017. *Radiology*. 2017;284(1):228–243.

Marotta G, Voltini F, Longari V, et al. FDG-PET and computed tomography in diagnosis of lung hamartoma. *J Nucl Med*. 2010;51(suppl 2): 1590.

Case 128

IN-111 OCTREOSCAN—MENINGIOMA

1. c
2. c
3. b
4. a

Discussion

This is an Octreoscan, which utilizes In-111 pentetreotide, a somatostatin receptor imaging radiopharmaceutical that is typically used to detect neuroendocrine tumors (i.e., carcinoid) but can also localize to non-neuroendocrine tumors that express somatostatin receptors (e.g., meningioma).

In this case, there is abnormal radiotracer uptake within the cranium to the left of midline. The location of the abnormal uptake makes a pituitary tumor less likely. Physiologic uptake may be seen in the pituitary, but usually it is not this intense. Expected physiologic uptake is seen in the liver, spleen, and kidneys, within the highest uptake in the spleen. The SPECT/CT shows an extra-axial mass, which demonstrates significant calcifications most compatible with a meningioma. We would not expect glioblastoma, metastases (carcinoid metastases to the brain are exceedingly rare), or meningitis to demonstrate significant increased uptake.

REFERENCES

Maini CL, Tofani A, Sciuto R, Carapella C, Cioffi R, Crecco M. Somatostatin receptors in meningiomas: a scintigraphic study using 111In-DTPA-D-Phe-1-octreotide. *Nucl Med Comm*. 1993;14(7):550–558.

Shi W, Johnston CF, Buchanan KD, et al. Localization of neuroendocrine tumours with [111In] DTPA-octreotide scintigraphy (Octreoscan): a comparative study with CT and MR imaging. *QJM*. 1998;91(4): 295–301.

Case 129

F-18 FLUCICLOVINE PET/CT (FACBC)

1. d
2. c
3. a
4. a

Discussion

Prostate cancer is the most prevalent cancer in men after lung cancer. Localizing disease in the setting of biochemical recurrence is a diagnostic dilemma. Metastatic disease may be present in nodes or bones that are not detected on conventional imaging studies (CT and MRI). F-18 FDG PET/CT has not proven to be valuable in the assessment of prostate cancer because of low utilization of glucose in prostate cancer. Other adenocarcinomas, such as lung and colon adenocarcinomas, have high uptake.

Several radiotracers have been introduced to localize disease in suspected metastatic prostate cancer. Some of the PET radio-pharmaceuticals include carbon-11 (C-11) choline, F-18 FACBC, and Ga-68 or F-18 prostate-specific membrane antigen (PSMA).

This case is an example of F-18 fluciclovine (Axumin®). This radiotracer was approved by the FDA in 2016. F-18 fluciclovine images demonstrate significant normal uptake in the pancreas, which receives the highest radiation dose. There is no significant uptake or clearance in the urinary system, which is of value when assessing the prostate gland. Further studies are needed to assess which one of the agents for the assessment of prostate cancer will be at the forefront. This study demonstrates a left common iliac node consistent with metastases. Focal uptake over the right upper lung zone on maximum-intensity projection (MIP) images proved to represent a right supraclavicular lymph node on cross-sectional imaging (not pictured).

REFERENCES

Turkbey B, Mena E, Shih J, et al. Localized prostate cancer detection with 18F FACBC PET/CT: comparison with MR imaging and histopathologic analysis. *Radiology*. 2013;270(3):849–856.

Shoup TM, Goodman MM. Synthesis of [F-18]-1-amino-3-fluoro-cyclobutane-1-carboxylic acid (FACBC): a PET tracer for tumor delineation. *J Labelled Comp Radiopharm*. 1999;42(3):215–225.

Case 130

F-18 FDG PET/CT—ERDHEIM-CHESTER DISEASE

1. a
2. b
3. c
4. b

Discussion

The F-18 FDG PET/CT scan shows increased FDG avidity in the distal femurs and proximal tibias, associated with CT-demonstrated patchy sclerosis of the medullary cavities.

Erdheim-Chester disease is a rare non-Langerhan's histiocytosis disease. The histiocytosis is characterized by infiltration of the skeleton and viscera by lipid-laden histiocytes, leading to fibrosis and osteosclerosis. There is some debate in the literature about this representing a reactive or neoplastic process. Erdheim-Chester disease affects multiple organ systems. The most common manifestation are bone lesions classically described as symmetric sclerosis involving the long tubular bones, most often in the metaphysis and diaphysis of the lower extremities. As well, Erdheim-Chester disease has a predilection for connective, adipose, and perivascular tissues. The soft tissue infiltration can extend throughout the length of the aorta and invade the retroperitoneum and the mediastinum, with potentially life-threatening complications such as heart failure, tamponade, and renal failure. Central nervous system involvement may include orbital, meningeal, and infundibular stalk masses, which may lead to exophthalmos and diabetes insipidus. F-18 FDG PET/CT offers the ability to evaluate for these multisystemic manifestations in a single imaging study. There is no standard treatment plan, with various treatments having limited success. Treatments include steroids, interferon, chemotherapy, radiation, and surgery.

REFERENCES

Steňová Emőke, et al. FDG-PET in the Erdheim–Chester disease: its diagnostic and follow-up role. *Rheumatol Int*. 2012;32(3):675–678.

Case 131

F-18 FDG PET/CT—TRANSVERSE MYELITIS

1. d
2. b
3. b
4. c

Discussion

This F-18 FDG PET/CT scan was performed to evaluate for underlying paraneoplastic disease in a patient with nonspecific neurologic complaints. The scan is an example of transverse myelitis, which is an inflammatory condition involving the cervical spinal cord. It tends to occur over multiple segments and cross the midline on axial images. This condition is best evaluated with MRI of the cervical spine. CT of the cervical spine will not adequately characterize conditions involving the spinal cord. CT myelography or biopsy would not be indicated until MRI is performed. In a patient with a recent history of immunization, the most likely diagnosis is transverse myelitis. The differential diagnosis includes tumors, demyelination, and acute disseminated encephalomyelitis (ADEM). The diagnosis cannot be made on FDG PET/CT alone. However, it is abnormal to have focal activity in the midcervical spinal cord. Possible etiologies include tumor, infection, and inflammation.

REFERENCES

Kamoto Y, Sadato N, Yonekura Y, et al. Visualization of the cervical spinal cord with FDG and high-resolution PET. *J Comput Assist Tomogr*. 1998;22(3):487–491.

Nguyen NC, Sayed MM, Taalab K, Osman MM. Spinal cord metastases from lung cancer: detection with F-18 FDG PET/CT. *Clin Nucl Med*. 2008;33(5):356–358.

Case 132

F-18 FDG PET—HERNIA PLUG STATUS POST HERNIA REPAIR

1. a
2. a
3. a
4. b

Discussion

Awareness of the imaging characteristics of an inguinal hernia plug is important when evaluating oncologic PET/CT scans. It is important not to mistake inflammatory changes from a surgical procedure for metastatic lymphadenopathy. Studies have shown that patients who had undergone an inguinal hernia plug repair showed increased FDG avidity associated with the plug on FDG PET/CT, whereas those who had undergone inguinal hernia mesh repair did not show hypermetabolic activity. Findings of increased uptake are likely related to inflammatory cells at the site of a foreign object. Uptake in the deep pelvis is related to physiologic bowel activity.

REFERENCES

Franceschi A, Friedman K, Ghesani M. Inguinal hernia repair mimicking cancer on PET-CT: mesh is cool, but the plug lights up. *J Nucl Med*. 2015;56(suppl 3): 1426.

Case 133

KARTAGENER'S SYNDROME

1. a
2. a
3. c
4. c

Discussion

This is a case of Kartagener's syndrome, characterized by dextrocardia with situs inversus, sinusitis, and bronchiectasis.

The axial CT image of the lungs demonstrates hypermetabolic inflammatory/infectious tubular mucus plugging within a dilated bronchus in the left upper lobe of the lung. Axial image of the sinuses shows maxillary sinus opacification consistent with sinusitis. MIP image from PET/CT illustrates dextrocardia with situs inversus.

This is an autosomal recessive inherited condition. Clinical symptoms are related to ciliary dysfunction, resulting in chronic infections of the ear, sinus, and lung caused by impaired mucus clearance. Infertility may occur in both males and females. Only 50% of patients with primary ciliary dyskinesia will have situs inversus. Treatment measures include aggressive treatment of the infection with antibiotics as well as aggressive physiotherapy for mucus clearance.

REFERENCES

Leigh MW, Pittman JE, Carson JL, et al. Clinical and genetic aspects of primary ciliary dyskinesia/Kartagener syndrome. *Genet Med*. 2009;11(7):473–487.

Ronnevi C, Ortiz-Villalon C, Pawlowski J, Ferrara G. Recurrent respiratory infections and unusual radiology: a woman with Kartagener's syndrome. *BMJ Case Rep*. 2015. Sep 9;2015. pii: bcr2015211650.https://doi.org/10.1136/bcr2015211650.

Case 134

F-18 FDG PET/CT—SINONASAL LYMPHOMA

1. a
2. c
3. c
4. d

Discussion

This case demonstrates an intensely avid mass in the anterior nares. This mass is solid, which is suggestive of a malignancy. Sinonasal malignancies are uncommon, accounting for less than 5% of head and neck malignancies. These malignancies encompass a variety of histologies, including squamous cell carcinoma, adenocarcinoma, esthesioneuroblastoma, lymphoma, and melanoma. Hence, treatment of sinonasal malignancies varies, depending on histology results. Sinonasal lymphoma is most frequently characterized as diffuse large B-cell lymphoma, followed by T-cell lymphoma. With primary sinonasal lymphoma, patients typically present with symptoms of rhinorrhea or paranasal sinus/nasal congestion. Because of its ability to provide exquisite soft tissue details, MRI is the best modality for the evaluation of locoregional disease.

REFERENCES

Cuadra-Garcia I, Proulx GM, Wu CL, et al. Sinonasal lymphoma: a clinicopathologic analysis of 58 cases from the Massachusetts General Hospital. *Am J Surg Pathol.* 1999;23(11):1356–1369.

Nicolai P, Castelnuovo P, Villaret AB. Endoscopic resection of sinonasal malignancies. *Curr Oncol Rep.* 2011;13(2):138–144.

Turner JH, Reh DD. Incidence and survival in patients with sinonasal cancer: A historical analysis of population-based data. *Head Neck.* 2012;34(6):877–885.

Vidal RW. Devaney K, Rinaldo A, Ferlito A, Carbone A. Sinonasal malignant lymphomas: a distinct clinicopathological category. *Ann Otol Rhinol Laryngol.* 1999;108(4):411–419.

Case 135

RENAL TC-99M SESTAMIBI SCAN

1. b
2. a
3. a
4. b

Discussion

The CT scan demonstrates a large, enhancing left renal mass with a central stellate scar. On the subsequent Tc-99m sestamibi SPECT/CT scan, this lesion demonstrates significant radiotracer uptake consistent with a benign entity of oncocytoma or oncocytoma/chromophobic adenoma. Most primary renal lesions represent renal cell carcinoma. However, up to 20% of renal lesions diagnosed on CT may represent a benign entity, such as oncocytoma, angiomyolipoma, or adenoma. The most common benign lesion is an oncocytoma. Because anatomic imaging cannot reliably distinguish between renal cell carcinoma and oncocytoma, many patients are subjected to invasive procedures, including biopsy and surgery for diagnosis. Approximately 5600 benign renal masses are resected in the United States each year.

Oncocytomas differ from other renal masses in that they are composed of a high number of mitochondria. Because of mitochondrial density, oncocytomas have significant Tc-99m sestamibi uptake on imaging. Multiple studies have found that Tc-99m sestamibi can reliably differentiate a benign lesion, such as oncocytoma, from malignant renal cell carcinoma, with a sensitivity of approximately 87% and a specificity of 95%.

REFERENCES

Gorin MA, Rowe SP, Baras AS, et al. Prospective evaluation of 99m Tc-sestamibi SPECT/CT for the diagnosis of renal oncocytomas and hybrid oncocytic/chromophobe tumors. *Eur Urol.* 2016;69(3): 413–416.

Gormley TS, Van Every MJ, Moreno AJ. Renal oncocytoma: preoperative diagnosis using technetium 99m sestamibi imaging. *Urology.* 1996;48(1):33–39.

Johnson DC, Vukina J, Smith AB, et al. Preoperatively misclassified, surgically removed benign renal masses: a systematic review of surgical series and United States population level burden estimate. *J Urol.* 2015;193(1):30–35.

Rowe SP, Gorin MA, Gordetsky J, et al. Initial experience using 99mTc-MIBI SPECT/CT for the differentiation of oncocytoma from renal cell carcinoma. *Clin Nucl Med.* 2015;40(4):309.

Case 136

I-131 UPTAKE IN A RENAL CYST

1. a
2. d
3. b
4. c

Discussion

This scan demonstrates poor body outline, suggesting considerable washout of radiopharmaceutical acquired a week after I-131 therapy. The artifact in the neck is related to the administered high dose and the high-energy I-131 dose penetrating the six-sided septa of the collimator (star artifact), also suggesting that it is a post-therapy scan. Finally, the liver is only seen on post-therapy scans, not pretherapy scans, because the administered high therapeutic dose allows one to see radiolabeled thyroxin metabolism in the liver. There is unexpected abnormal focal uptake in the left abdomen that does not conform to the expected anatomy of the bowel. Bowel activity seen on I-131 scans is physiologic, but not always present a week after therapy. The SPECT/CT scan demonstrates that the radioactivity is within a renal cyst, and this is confirmed by ultrasonography. Clearance via a hydronephrotic collecting system would look similar on the I-131 scan. Other cystic structures, including ovarian, breast, thymic, hepatic, and bronchogenic cysts, rarely may also accumulate the radiotracer. Although the exact mechanism for this occurrence is not known, it is hypothesized that entry is by passive diffusion or active transport where the tracer becomes trapped.

REFERENCES

Bakheet SM, Hammami MM, Powe J. False-positive radioiodine uptake in the abdomen and the pelvis: radioiodine retention in the kidneys and review of the literature. *Clin Nucl Med.* 1996;21(12):932–937.

Kraft O, Širucek P, Mrhac L, Havel M. I-131 false positive uptake in a huge parapelvic renal cyst. *Nucl Med Rev.* 2011;14(1):36–37.

Oh JR, Ahn BC. False-positive uptake on radioiodine whole-body scintigraphy: physiologic and pathologic variants unrelated to thyroid cancer. *Am J Nucl Med Mol Imaging.* 2012;2(3):362.

Case 137

GASTRIC CARCINOID

1. c
2. b
3. a
4. a

Discussion

Abnormal increased In-111 Octreoscan uptake is seen in the stomach on this study. In addition, on SPECT/CT images, there is a lesion adjacent to the head of the pancreas. Findings are compatible with somatostatin receptor–positive tissue. This patient has a history of multiple endocrine neoplasia type 1 (MEN1) and a prior resection of a gastrinoma. Repeat surgery revealed a recurrent gastrinoma adjacent to the pancreas, as well as numerous gastric carcinoid tumors likely related to increased gastrin levels.

Gastric carcinoids are thought to be rare tumors. There are three types of gastric carcinoids. The most common gastric carcinoid is type I. It is closely associated with chronic atrophic gastritis. Type II gastric carcinoid is associated with MEN1 and Zollinger-Ellison syndrome. Type III gastric carcinoid is thought to behave more aggressively than types I and II.

REFERENCES

Nikou George C, Angelopoulos Theodoros P. Current concepts on gastric carcinoid tumors. *Gastroenterol Res Pract.* 2012;2012:287825.

Öberg K, Eriksson B. Nuclear medicine in the detection, staging and treatment of gastrointestinal carcinoid tumours. *Best Pract Res Clin Endocrinol Metab.* 2005;19(2):265–276.

Case 138

F-18 FDG PET/CT—MULTIPLE SCLEROSIS

1. a
2. a
3. b
4. d

Discussion

The F-18 FDG PET/CT scan shows rounded FDG-avid lesions in the white matter bilaterally, largest in the right frontoparietal region with incomplete peripheral ring activity. The concurrent contrast-enhanced MRI of the brain demonstrates an incomplete, peripherally enhancing lesion. The presence of Dawson's fingers (demyelinating lesions orientate perpendicular to the ventricles/along the medullary veins) on MRI is compatible with the diagnosis of multiple sclerosis (MS).

MS is a neurodegenerative disease that manifests itself as demyelination and active inflammation in the central nervous system. The characteristic histology finding are demyelinating lesions. Foci of increased FLAIR/T2 signal on MRI of the brain that are orientated perpendicular to the length of the lateral ventricles are characteristic of the disease and referred to as *Dawson's fingers*. FDG PET/CT is not routinely used for the evaluation of MS. However, lesions may demonstrate increased F-18 FDG uptake in patients being evaluated for other reasons. Increased activity is thought to be related to active inflammation. Although FDG PET can detect active inflammation, the high background physiologic cortical activity in the brain often limits the clinical utility of this radiotracer. Further investigations are need to assess the clinical utility of new radiotracers, for example, those targeting inflammation or myelination/demyelination specifically.

REFERENCE

Olivero WC, Dulebohn SC, Lister JR. The use of PET in evaluating patients with primary brain tumours: is it useful? *J Neurol Neurosurg Psychiatry*. 1995;58(2):250–252.

Case 139

LUMBOPERITONEAL SHUNT PATENCY EVALUATION

1. a
2. a
3. b
4. c

Discussion

On the prior study, the patient had symptoms of increasing headache and poor balance. The radiotracer is injected intrathecally for this lumboperitoneal shunt study. The prior study (image A) demonstrates radiotracer activity within the spinal column only. This is a nonfunctioning shunt. The shunt was corrected, and now similar symptoms have recurred; however, this study (image B) shows that the shunt is functioning with flow into the peritoneum. There are many types of cerebrospinal fluid (CSF) diversion shunts to treat communicating and noncommunicating hydrocephalus. These include ventriculoperitoneal (VP) shunts, ventriculoatrial (VA) shunts, ventriculopleural (VPl) shunts, and lumboperitoneal (LP) shunts. LP shunts are uncommon, usually placed when other shunts have malfunctioned. Shunt studies are performed when the patient presents with symptoms of shunt malfunction, which cannot be definitely assessed on clinical examination. Shunts should be accessed with aseptic technique by a professional who is familiar with the specific shunt type. When using Tc-99m diethylenetriamine penta-acetic acid (DTPA), typically 1 mCi is injected into the shunt reservoir or the subarachnoid space for LP shunts. This tracer is not FDA approved for CSF studies so this would be off label use of the radiotracer. In-111 DTPA may also be used, but this tracer is expensive, and its long half-life is not required for this particular study. VP, VA, and VPl shunt assessment images demonstrate activity originating in the cranium, whereas LP shunt evaluation images demonstrate activity only within the distal spinal column. A high accuracy for the test has been reported.

REFERENCES

El-Saadany WF, Farhoud A, Zidan I. Lumboperitoneal shunt for idiopathic intracranial hypertension: patients' selection and outcome. *Neurosurg Rev.* 2012;35(2):239–244.

Graham P, Howman-Giles R, Johnston I, Besser M. Evaluation of CSF shunt patency by means of technetium-99m DTPA. *J Neurosurg.* 1982;57(2):262–266.

Yadav Y, Pande S, Raina V, Singh M. Lumboperitoneal shunts: review of 409 cases. *Neurol India.* 2004;52(2):188.

Case 140

LAMINAR NECROSIS

1. b
2. a
3. a
4. d

Discussion

This is a case of focal uptake within the brain parenchyma on a bone scan. Extraosseous uptake in the brain is a rare occurrence (<1% of cases) on bone scans. On the planar images, it is not clear whether this uptake is in the brain parenchyma or in the skull. SPECT/CT clearly localizes this activity to the brain parenchyma. Physiologic activity in the brain is not seen on normal bone scans. There are several possible etiologies for abnormal uptake in the brain on bone scans. These include tumors, infarctions, encephalitis, and recent surgery. Uptake in the setting of brain infarctions is thought to be related to influx of calcium into the damaged neurons as a result of cell membrane dysfunction. This leads to intracellular calcium precipitates. Radiotracer uptake will reflect the extent of neuronal damage. In this case, as noted on subsequent MRI of the brain, (images C & D) findings were consistent with cortical laminar necrosis. This typically occurs in the setting of hypoxia, hypoglycemia, cardiac arrest, and status epilepticus. It is caused by the inability to maintain oxygenation or glucose demand in the cortices. The hallmark of laminar necrosis on MRI is T1 cortical hyperintensity. Later on, this may be associated with enhancement.

REFERENCES

Gentili A, Miron SD, Bellon EM. Nonosseous accumulation of bone-seeking radiopharmaceuticals. *Radiographics*. 1990;10(5):871–881.

Kannivelu A, Padhy AK, Srinivasan S, Ali SZ. Extraosseous uptake of technetium-99m methylene diphosphonate by an acute territorial cerebral infarct in a classical biodistribution pattern. *Indian J Nucl Med*. 2013;28(4) 240.

Mackie GC. Tc-99m MDP uptake resulting from acute middle cerebral artery territory infarction. *Clin Nucl Med*. 2003;28(10):851–852.

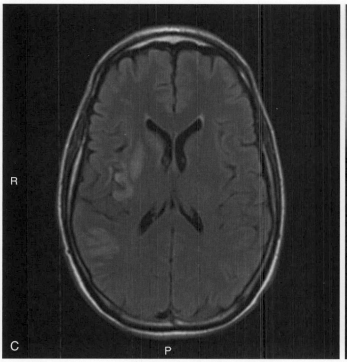

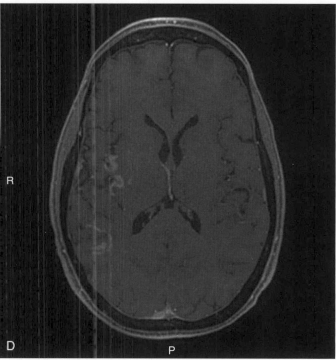

Case 141

F-18 FDG PET/CT ULCERATIVE COLITIS "LEAD PIPE" SIGN

1. a
2. c
3. b
4. b

Discussion

This case demonstrates a featureless rectosigmoid colon—the "lead pipe" sign. This is seen in patients with ulcerative colitis (UC).

Patients with UC tend to be young at diagnosis, less than 40 years of age, and typically present with relapsing bloody diarrhea. UC is an inflammatory condition that involves the mucosa and submucosa of the colon, beginning in the rectum, with proximal continuous extension to part or all of the colon. The "lead pipe" sign is thought to be caused by hypertrophy of the muscularis mucosa. The patients are at increased risk of malignancy. Therapy is dictated by extent of disease and severity of symptoms. Medical therapy, which may include sulfasalazine, steroids, immunosuppressives, and biologics, is directed at reducing inflammation. However, for those with severe disease and intractable symptoms, surgery may be indicated.

The CT finding on this study is diagnostic. This finding might be found incidentally on a PET/CT scan. F-18 FDG PET/CT may be beneficial as adjunct tests when colonoscopy yields incomplete results or other tests are inconclusive. FDG PET/CT may be utilized for evaluation of malignancy in high-risk patients. Although this technique may also be utilized for evaluation of underlying inflammation and therapy efficacy, it is significantly hampered by normal physiologic bowel activity, which may have a similar metabolic profile to inflamed colonic mucosa. Radiolabeled leukocytes can also be utilized for confirming active disease, localization, and response to therapy.

REFERENCE

Perlman SB, Hall BS, Reichelderfer M. PET/CT imaging of inflammatory bowel disease. In: *Seminars in Nuclear Medicine*. Vol. 43. No. 6.WB Saunders; 2013:420–426.

Case 142

BRAIN INTERICTAL/ICTAL SPECT

1. d
2. b
3. a
4. a

Discussion

This case demonstrates relative photopenia in the left temporal lobe on an interictal scan and relative increased uptake in the same region on an ictal study. In a patient with a history of seizures, these findings would be compatible with a seizure focus. Patients with complex partial seizures refractory to medical therapy may greatly benefit from surgical resection. Hence, exact localization of the seizure focus is paramount. Surgical intervention of temporal lobe abnormalities may result in marked improvement in 80% of patients. A multipronged approach for localizing seizure foci is employed, including thorough neurologic examination, EEG, CT/MRI, and molecular imaging. Invasive techniques utilizing depth electrodes may also be used. The constellation of findings is then summarized to decide whether surgery will be beneficial.

Nuclear medicine techniques for seizure localization may include gamma camera or PET imaging. An ictal study is performed with either Tc-99m ethyl cysteinate dimer (ECD) or HMPAO. Patients are admitted to a monitoring unit (video and EEG) so that the radiotracer can be injected within 1 to 2 minutes of seizure onset. Generally, the radiotracer is stored at the bedside in a lead box. Because the radiotracer after injection is trapped within the neuron, imaging can be delayed up to several hours. A baseline interictal SPECT is obtained to assess for a mismatch. Classically, the interictal SPECT will show a photopenic defect, although at times the focus may be isointense to the adjacent brain parenchyma and therefore difficult to identify. Interictal PET is likely a better study to identify a seizure focus, also demonstrating a photopenic defect. The ictal SPECT will demonstrate a focus of increased activity above that of adjacent brain parenchyma. Ictal F-18 FDG PET scans are generally not performed because of the short half-life of F-18, which renders the study impractical. On occasion, one may see an ictal FDG PET if the patient has an incidental seizure during the uptake period. Hence, the most sensitive scintigraphic technique for identifying seizure foci is a combination of ictal SPECT and interictal PET scan.

REFERENCES

Oliveira AJ, Costa JC, Hilário LN, Anselmi OE, Palmini A. Localization of the epileptogenic zone by ictal and interictal SPECT with 99mTc-ethyl cysteinate dimer in patients with medically refractory epilepsy. *Epilepsia.* 1999;40(6):693–702.

Tae WS, Joo EY, Kim JH, et al. Cerebral perfusion changes in mesial temporal lobe epilepsy: SPM analysis of ictal and interictal SPECT. *Neuroimage.* 2005;24(1):101–110.

Case 143

VENTILATION SCAN—BRONCHOPLEURAL FISTULA

1. a
2. d
3. a
4. d

Discussion

This study shows the xenon-133 (Xe-133) gas being inhaled and then exhaled. It is seen in the pneumonectomy cavity clearing through the pleural effusion drainage catheter, evidence of a bronchopleural fistula. Xe-133 is well suited for this examination because it is a dynamic study showing the inhalation and exhalation of the gas. A Tc-99m DTPA aerosol study would not be useful because the aerosol particles impact and are retained in the alveoli. A bronchopleural fistula is an abnormal communication between the bronchial tree and the pleura. The most common cause is prior lung resection. Less common causes include lung necrosis related to infection, prior chemotherapy or radiation to the lung fields, pleuroparenchymal fibroelastosis, and persistent pneumothorax. The diagnosis may be suggested on the basis of such findings as increase in intrapleural air, new hydropneumothorax, or pneumomediastinum on chest imaging. The Xe-133 ventilation study is confirmatory.

REFERENCE

Nielsen KR, Blake LM, Mark JB, DeCampli W, McDougall IR. Localization of bronchopleural fistula using ventilation scintigraphy. *J Nucl Med*. 1994;35(5):867–869.

Case 144

BONE SCAN—MASTOIDITIS/MALIGNANT EXTERNAL OTITIS

1. a
2. b
3. a
4. b

Discussion

Malignant external otitis is a serious and potentially life-threatening condition caused by an infection by *Pseudomonas*. This diagnosis is most commonly seen in the setting of diabetes mellitus. The three-phase planar bone scan demonstrates increased uptake on all three phases in the region of the temporal bone/mastoids. Only the delayed images are shown. The SPECT/CT better localizes the abnormal uptake. Ga-67 and In-111 leukocytes imaging can also be employed for diagnosis and would be particularly useful for assessing treatment response.

REFERENCES

Rubin J, Victor LY. Malignant external otitis: insights into pathogenesis, clinical manifestations, diagnosis, and therapy. *Am J Med*. 1988;85(3):391–398.

Strashun AM, Nejatheim M, Goldsmith SJ. Malignant external otitis: early scintigraphic detection. *Radiology*. 1984;150(2):541–545.

Case 145

RENAL EN BLOC

1. c
2. a
3. b
4. b

Discussion

This is a case of renal en bloc transplantation. It is the transplantation of two pediatric kidneys into the right or left lower quadrant. The native aorta and the inferior vena cava are anastomosed to the external iliac artery and vein. Given the increasing need for renal transplantation, transplants from pediatric donors have been explored in an effort to increase the number of available organs. Donors tend to be less than 5 years of age. The most common cause for graft failure is thought to be vascular dysfunction. Renal en bloc transplants are also prone to complications that are common to single adult renal transplants. It is important to evaluate each kidney during a renal scan. The United Network of Organ Sharing (UNOS) concluded that en bloc transplantation of renal transplants from young patients (<5 years of age) is a good alternative to single adult renal transplants.

REFERENCES

Dharnidharka VR, Stevens G, Howard RJ. En-bloc kidney transplantation in the United States: an analysis of United Network of Organ Sharing (UNOS) data from 1987 to 2003. *Am J Transplant.* 2005;5(6):1513–1517.

Mwipatayi BP, Leong CW, Subramanian P, Picardo A. En bloc kidney transplant from an 18-month-old donor to an adult recipient: case report and literature review. *Int J Surg Case Rep.* 2013;4(11): 948–951.

Case 146

GALLIUM-67 SEPTIC JOINT/OSTEOMYELITIS

1. d
2. a
3. c
4. b

Discussion

This Ga-67 citrate scan was performed for the evaluation of fever and left knee pain. There is focal abnormal uptake in the region of the left knee. A follow-up plain film of the left knee demonstrates an effusion. Findings are consistent with a septic joint. There is also focal uptake in the proximal left tibia consistent with osteomyelitis. Ga-67 is injected intravenously. It binds to transferrin in plasma. The primary gamma photon peaks are 93, 184, 296, and 388 keV. An easy way to remember the peaks is to round the numbers up or down to approximately 90, 190, 290, and 390 keV. Ga-67 initially is excreted via the kidneys and subsequently through the intestine. This agent has traditionally been used to evaluate for infection/inflammation and tumors (i.e., lymphoma). Because of advanced techniques, Ga-67 is not really utilized for the evaluation of tumors today, but many clinics routinely use whole-body Ga-67 imaging for the evaluation of an underlying infectious process. The ideal imaging time for the evaluation of infections is 24 hours after injection. Bowel uptake limits the utility of this technique for the evaluation of abdominal infectious processes. SPECT/CT can be helpful in selected cases. If there is a clinical concern about an intraabdominal abscess, an In-111 WBC scan should be performed.

REFERENCE

Palestro CJ. The current role of gallium imaging in infection. In: *Seminars in Nuclear Medicine*. Vol. 24. No. 2. WB Saunders; 1994:128–141.

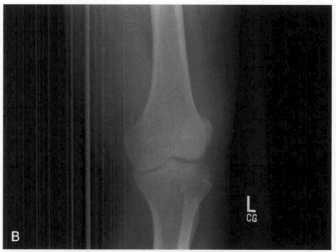

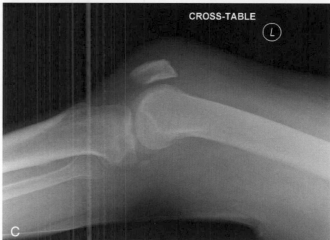

Case 147

RADIOACTIVE MATERIAL SPILLS

1. c
2. a
3. b
4. b

Discussion

Radioactive spills may occur at any facility. These are classically defined as major or minor based on dosage and radionuclide. Instructions on how to handle spills should be readily available and in clear sight at every site. In the event of a minor spill, persons in the area should be alerted to the occurrence, and the spill should be contained by using absorbent paper. Protective clothing should be worn during containment. Subsequently, the area as well as the personnel involved in the clean up of the spill should be surveyed. The incident should be reported to the radiation safety officer (RSO). In the event of a major spill, the RSO must be notified immediately, and the area must be cleared of patients and nonessential personnel and secured from entry by nonessential personnel. The spill must be contained by using absorbent paper but should not be cleaned up. Shielding of the

TABLE 147.1	
Radionuclide	**Major Spill Threshold**
Technetium-99m	100 mCi
Thallium-201	100 mCi
Gallium-67	10 mCi
Iodine-123	10 mCi
Indium-111	10 mCi
Cobalt-57	10 mCi
Iodine-131	1 mCi

site should be considered. Decontamination of personnel must be performed. A report to the Nuclear Regulatory Commission (NRC) may be required. The thresholds for major and minor spills for common radionuclides are listed above.

REFERENCES

Cherry SR, Sorenson JA, Phelps ME. *Physics in Nuclear Medicine E-Book.* Elsevier Health Sciences; 2012.

Ziessman HA, O'Malley JP, Thrall JH. *Nuclear Medicine: The Requisites E-Book.* Elsevier Health Sciences; 2013.

Case 148

TRANSPORTATION

1. b
2. d
3. c
4. a

Discussion

The above image is an example of labels required on packages containing radionuclides. All Nuclear Medicine departments receive radionuclides from outside entities, whether in the form of single-use or multiple-use doses or generators. All packages must be labeled with one of the following three categories:

Radioactive I: No special handling. Surface dose rate must not exceed 0.5 mrem/hr.

Radioactive II: Special handling. Surface dose rate must not exceed 50 mrem/hr and 1 mrem/hr at 1 m.

Radioactive III: Special handling. Surface dose rate must not exceed 200 mrem/hr and 10 mrem/hr at 1 m. Must be greater than 50 mrem/hr at the surface.

The label should also display which radionuclide is being transported under content as well as the activity of said radionuclide. Once these packages are received in the Nuclear Medicine department, they must be stored in a safe and secure place. The receipt of the package must be properly documented in a log. These logs must be maintained in case of an inspection by an internal or external authority. Packages that must be monitored must be assessed within 3 hours of receipt or, if received after hours, within 3 hours of the next business day opening.

REFERENCE

Ziessman HA, O Malley JP, Thrall JH. *Nuclear Medicine: The Requisites*. E-Book. Elsevier Health Sciences; 2013.

Case 149

PROSTATE CANCER IMAGING—F-18 PSMA PET/CT

1. c
2. b
3. d
4. a

Discussion

The images shown are from a F-18 PSMA scan. The radiopharmaceutical binds to PSMA, which is overexpressed on prostate cancer cells. Prostate cancer cells are not the only cells that express PSMA. Physiologic uptake is seen in salivary glands and kidneys because of increased numbers of PSMA antigens. Similar biodistribution is seen with Ga-68– and Tc-99m–labeled PSMA agents. Small deposits of disease can be detected because of the high antigen expression and resulting high tumor-to-background ratios.

Prostate cancer is the most common malignancy and a leading cause of cancer-related deaths in men. Several novel PET imaging agents have been investigated, including F-18 FACBC, C-11 choline, and Ga-68/F-18 PSMA, to name a few. C-11 Pittsburg compound B (PiB) binds to amyloid and has been used in the evaluation of Alzheimer's disease. NaF is a bone imaging radiopharmaceutical. Ga-68 DOTA-TATE is a somatostatin receptor neuroendocrine tumor–imaging agent. Better imaging techniques are being explored, as conventional imaging (CT/MRI) modalities often do not identify disease sites in patients with biochemical recurrence and small deposits. Data have shown that these novel PET agents are superior to conventional CT and MRI for detection of primary disease as well as regional and distant metastases. Early diagnosis with early intervention may lead better outcomes. Lutetium-177 (Lu-177)–labeled PSMA has been used as a therapeutic agent in Europe with encouraging results.

REFERENCES

Rowe SP, Macura KJ, Mena E, et al. PSMA-based [18F] DCFPyL PET/CT is superior to conventional imaging for lesion detection in patients with metastatic prostate cancer. *Mol Imaging Biol.* 2016;18(3):411–419.

Szabo Z, Mena E, Rowe SP, et al. Initial evaluation of [18F] DCFPyL for prostate-specific membrane antigen (PSMA)-targeted PET imaging of prostate cancer. *Mol Imaging Biol.* 2015;17(4):565–574.

Index of Cases

Note: Page numbers followed by "f" indicate figures and "t" indicate tables.

Index of Terms

Note: Page numbers followed by "f" indicate figures and "t" indicate tables.